Pharmaceutical Formulation Design - Recent Practices

Edited by Usama Ahmad and Juber Akhtar

Published in London, United Kingdom

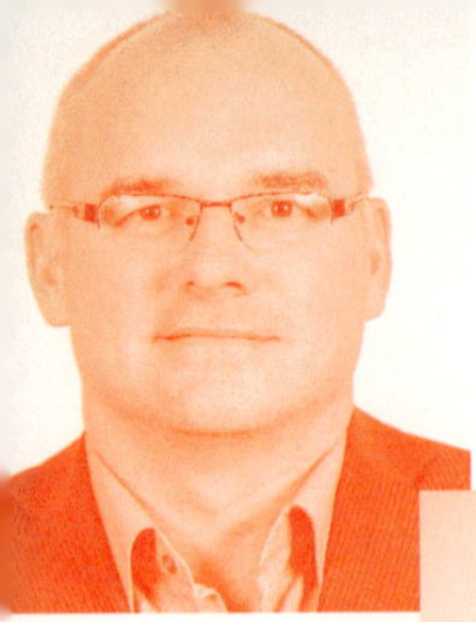
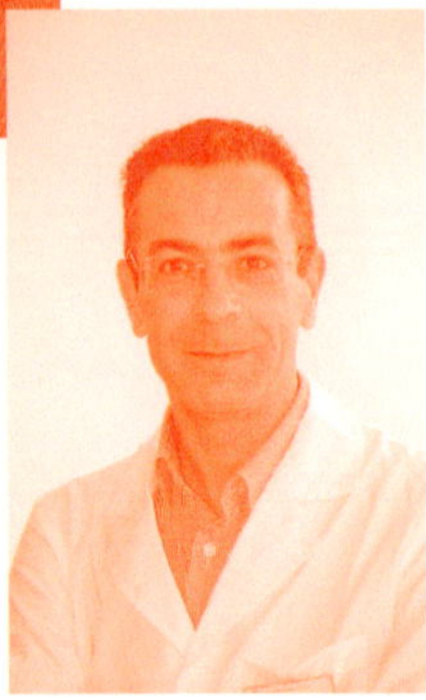
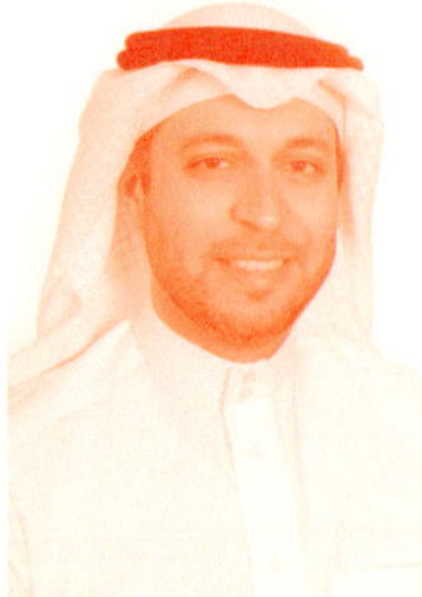
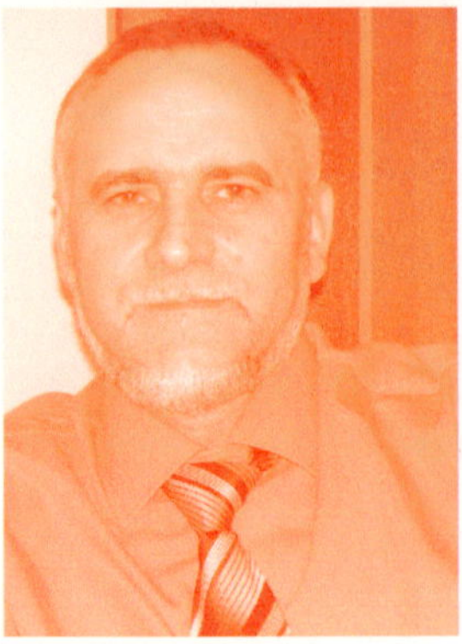
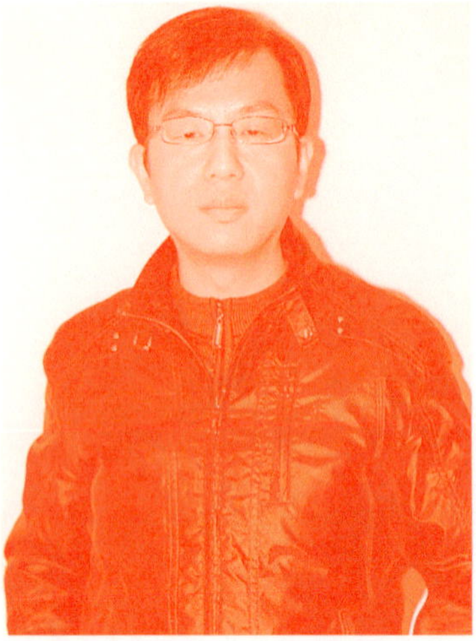
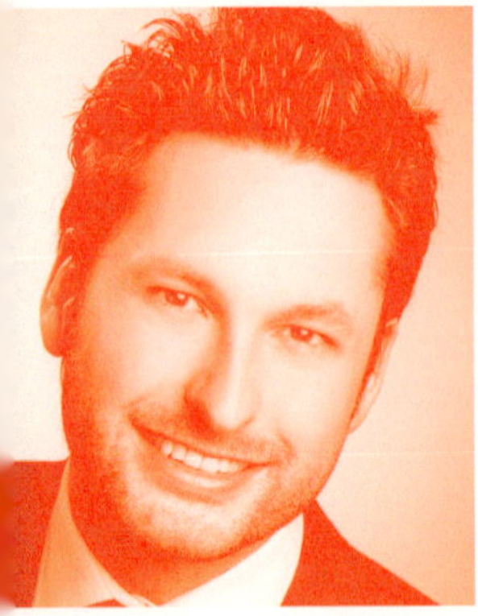
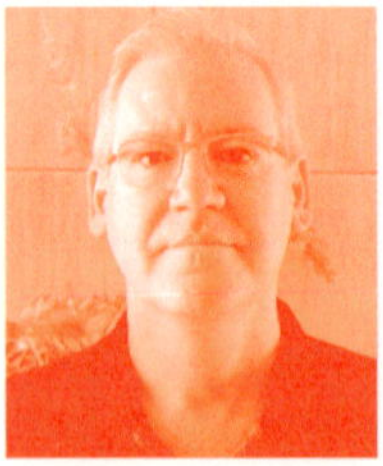

IntechOpen

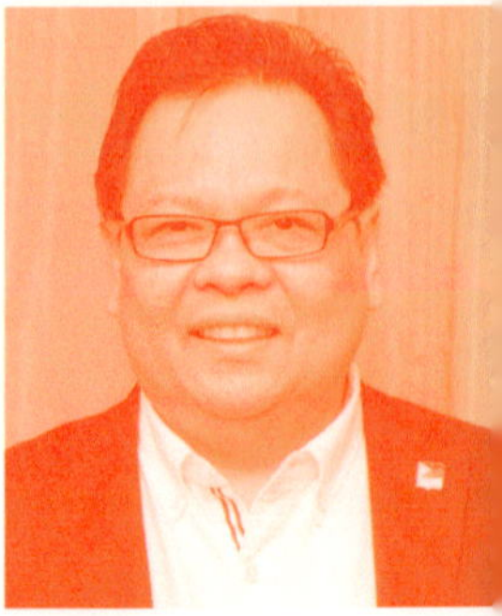
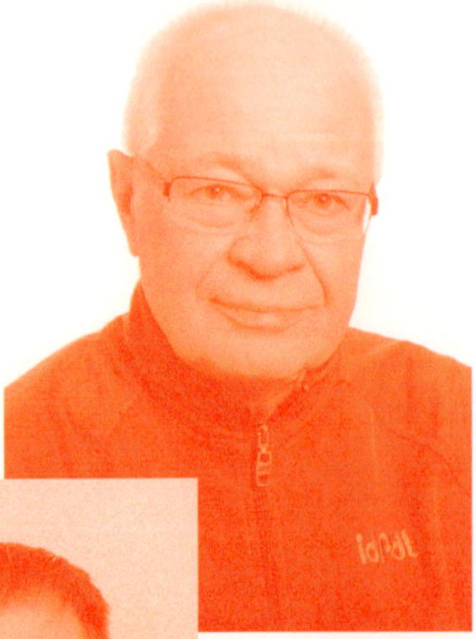
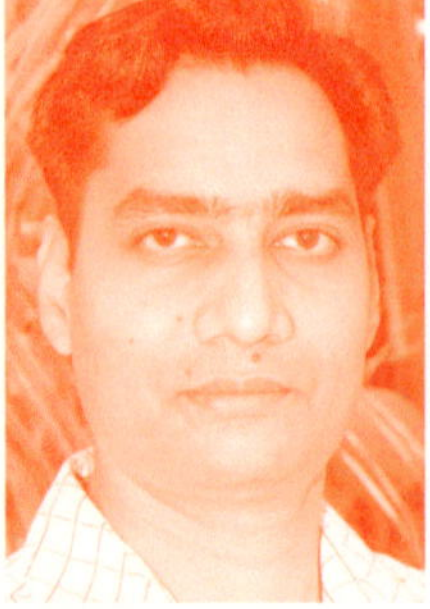
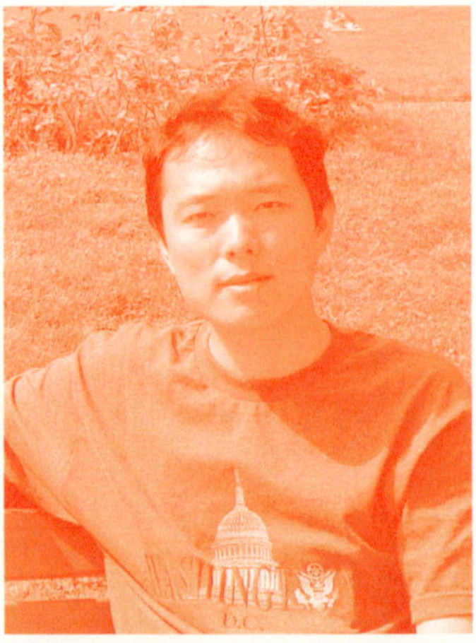
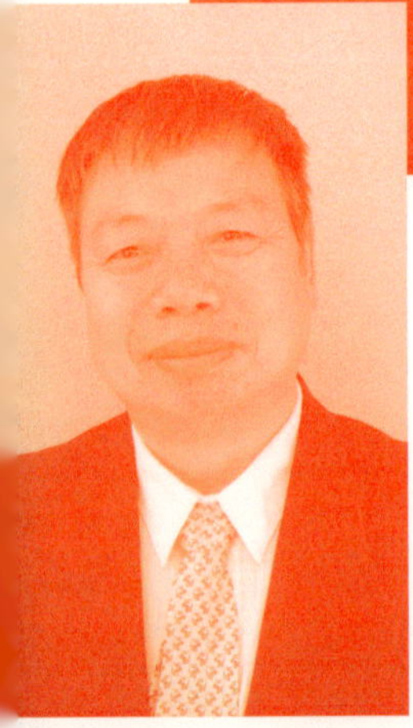
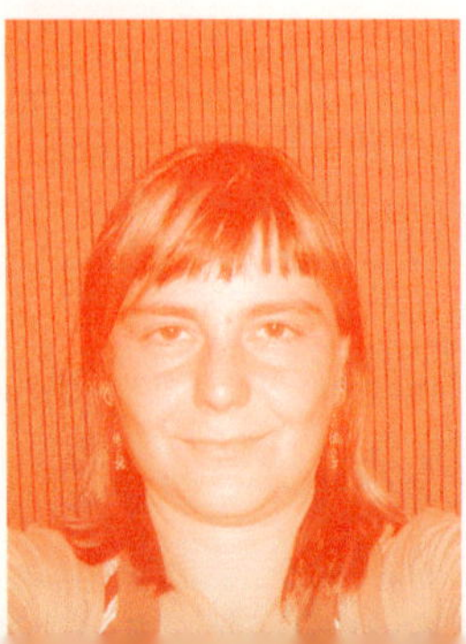

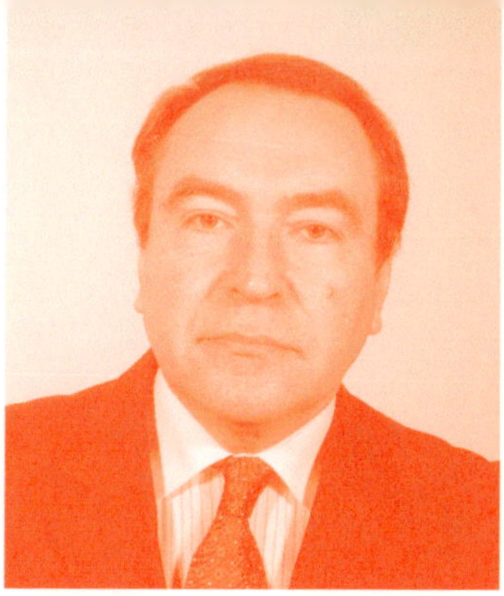

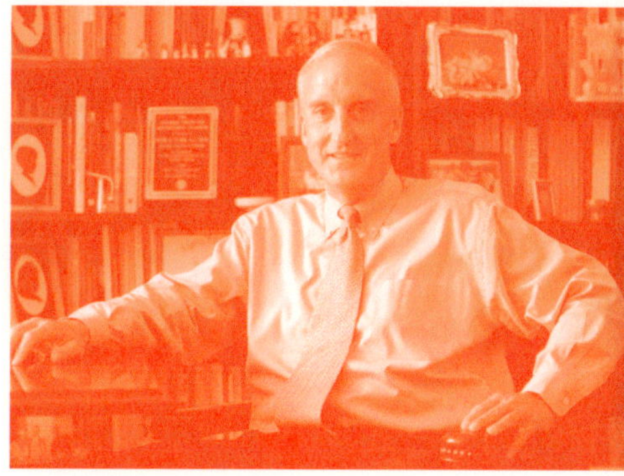

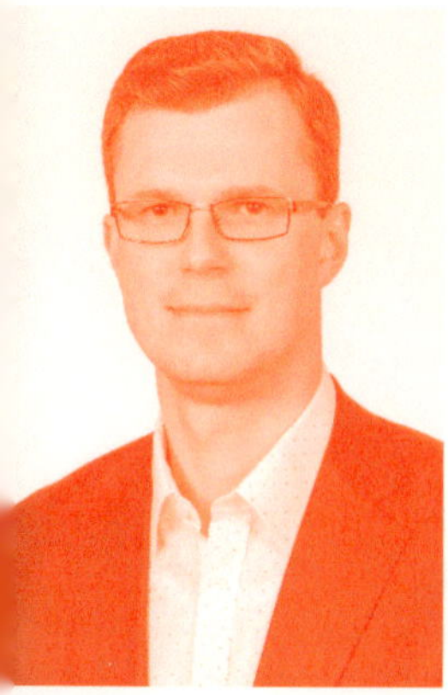

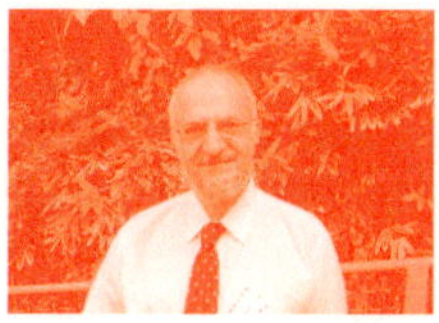

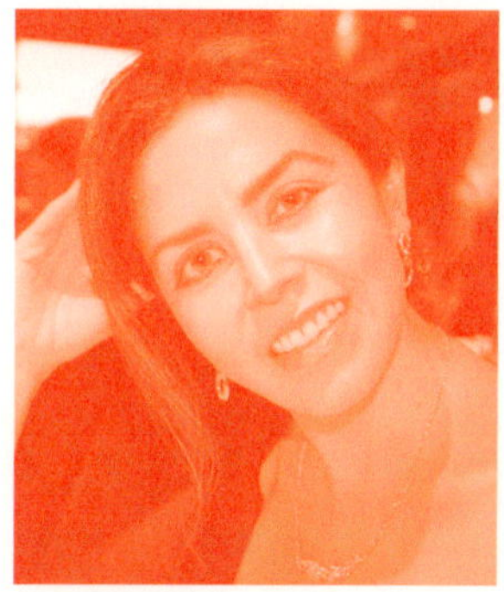

Supporting open minds since 2005

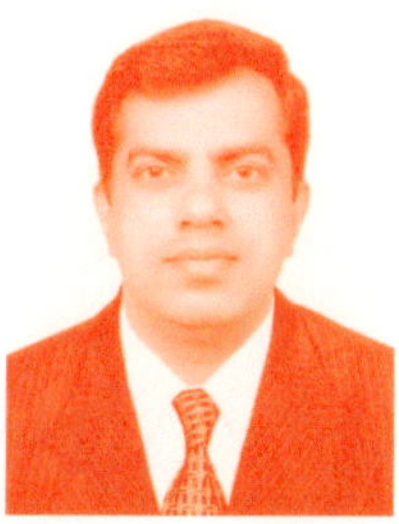

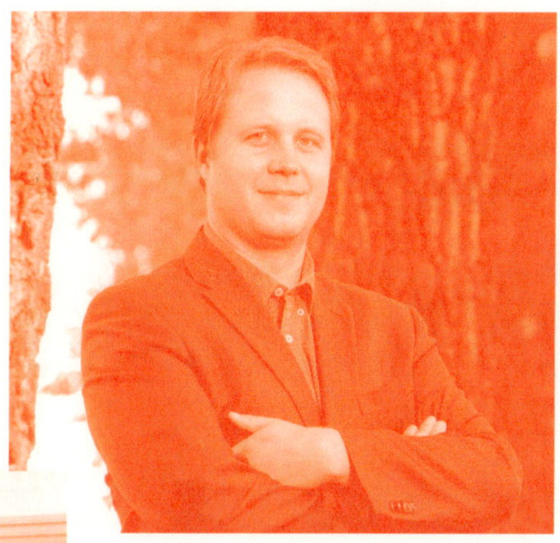

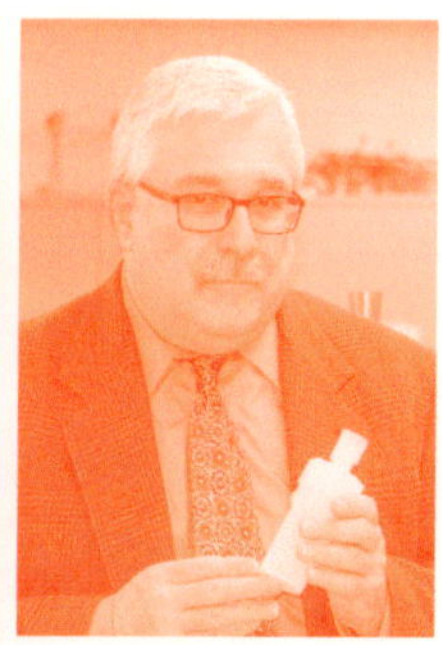

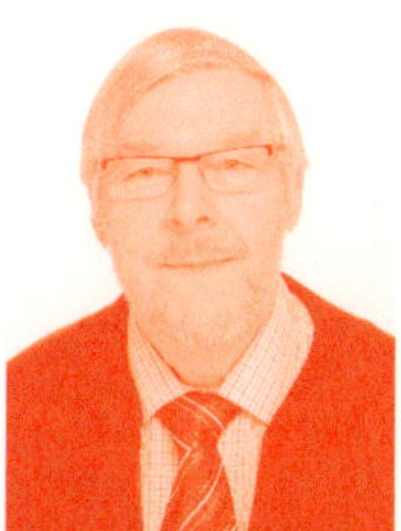

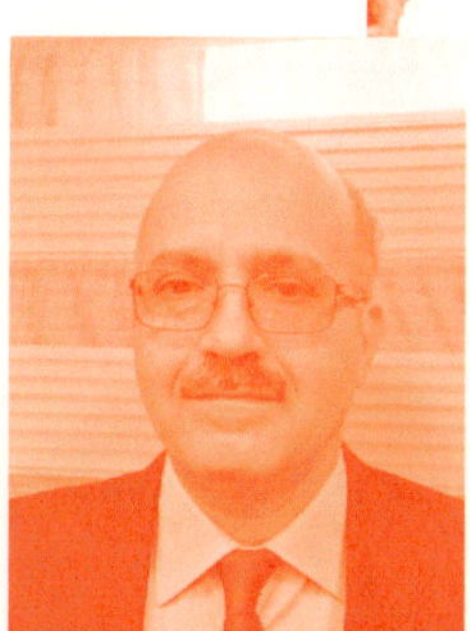

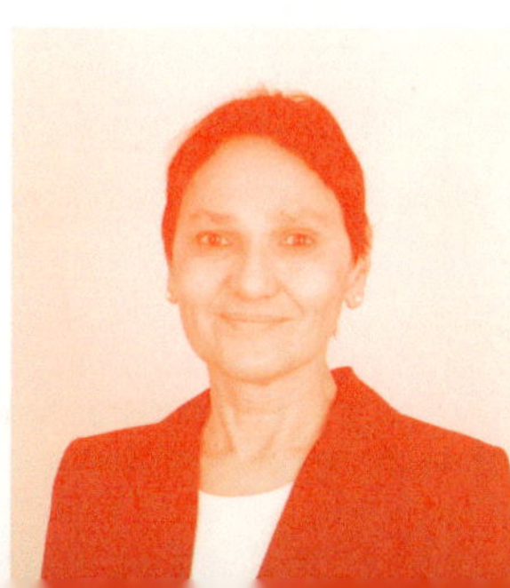

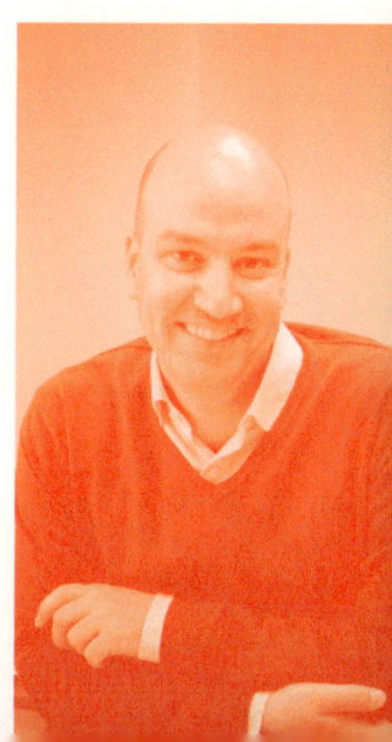

Pharmaceutical Formulation Design - Recent Practices
http://dx.doi.org/10.5772/intechopen.78460
Edited by Usama Ahmad and Juber Akhtar

Contributors
Shaza Shantier, Zermina Rashid, Pinak Patel, Anis Yohana Chaerunisaa, Marline Abdassah, Sriwidodo Sriwidodo, Harsha Virsingh Sonaye, Chandrashekhar Doifode, Mohmad Rafik Yakub Shaikh, Mahira Zeeshan, Mahwash Mukhtar, Hussain Ali, Qurat Ul Ain, Salman Khan, Hema Naga Durga, Usama Ahmad

First published in London, United Kingdom, 2020 by IntechOpen
IntechOpen is the global imprint of INTECHOPEN LIMITED, registered in England and Wales, registration number: 11086078, 7th floor, 10 Lower Thames Street, London, EC3R 6AF, United Kingdom
Printed in Croatia

British Library Cataloguing-in-Publication Data
A catalogue record for this book is available from the British Library

Additional hard and PDF copies can be obtained from orders@intechopen.com

Pharmaceutical Formulation Design - Recent Practices
Edited by Usama Ahmad and Juber Akhtar
p. cm.
Print ISBN 978-1-78985-662-0
Online ISBN 978-1-78985-839-6
eBook (PDF) ISBN 978-1-78985-840-2

Meet the editors

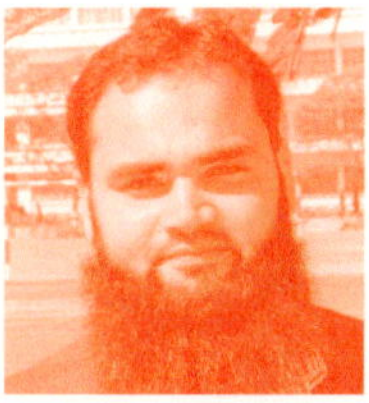

Dr Usama Ahmad holds a specialization in pharmaceutics from Amity University, Lucknow, India. He received his Ph.D. degree from Integral University on the work titled 'Development and evaluation of silymarin nanoformulation for hepatic carcinoma'. Currently, he's working as an Assistant Professor of Pharmaceutics at the Faculty of Pharmacy, Integral University. He has been teaching Pharm. D, B. Pharm, and M. Pharm students and conducting research in the novel drug delivery domain. From 2013 to 2014 he worked on a research project funded by SERB-DST, Government of India. He has rich publication records with more than fifteen original articles published in reputed journals, one book chapter with McGraw Hill Publishers, and a number of scientific articles published in 'Ingredients South Asia Magazine' and 'QualPharma Magazine'. He is a member of the American Association for Cancer Research, Commonwealth Pharmacist Association, and British Society for Nanomedicine. Dr Ahmad's research focus is on the development of nanoformulations to facilitate the delivery of drugs to provide practical solutions to current healthcare problems.

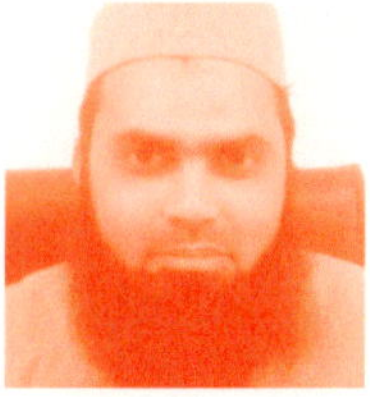

Dr Juber Akhtar completed his B. Pharm in 2005 from Jamia Hamdard University, New Delhi. In 2007 he completed his M. Pharm with specialization in Pharmaceutics from Manipal University, Karnataka. He obtained his PhD degree from Integral University in 2014. He is currently employed as an Associate Professor at Integral University. He acted as Head of Department from 2014 to 2016. He has experience in teaching abroad and has served as a Professor at Buraydah College of Dentistry and Pharmacy, KSA. Dr Akhtar has more than 40 publications in reputed journals and is also an editorial member of many esteemed journals. He has supervised a dozen PhD and M. Pharm students in research projects. Dr Akhtar is actively involved in research activities and his areas of interest include development of a nano particulate drug delivery system to target various organs.

Contents

Preface

Pharmaceutical formulations have evolved from simple and traditional systems to more modern and complex novel dosage forms. Formulation development is a tedious process and requires an enormous amount of effort from many different people. Developing a stable novel dosage form and further targeting it to the desired site inside the body has always been a challenge. The purpose of this book is to bring together scholarly articles that highlight recent developments and trends in pharmaceutical formulation science. Each article has been written by authors specializing in the subject area and hailing from top institutions around the world. The entire book has been written in a systematic and lucid style explaining all basic concepts and fundamentals in a very simple way.

Developing a novel dosage form necessitates the formulators to possess sound knowledge of preformulation studies. Prior to developing a stable formulation, knowledge and estimation of various physicochemical properties of the drug is a necessity. Estimation of drug solubility, partition coefficient, melting point etc. helps in selecting a proper route and dosage form for the drug. For this reason, a chapter is solely dedicated to preformulation studies and this will not only help the investigators but also students of pharmaceutics developing novel dosage forms. A chapter on drug analysis describes the different techniques and instruments used for identification and analysis of drugs in biological samples and formulations. Techniques such as UV spectrophotometry, derivative and difference spectrophotometry, chromatographic methods such as HPLC, HPTLC etc. are described in detail. Estimation of bioavailability of a drug is crucial in pharmaceutical sciences as it's the amount of drug that is available in systemic circulation to show its therapeutic efficacy. The chapter on bioavailability and bioequivalence highlights the strategies employed in designing experiments for conducting bioavailability and bioequivalence studies along with the methods used for estimation of drug concentration. A very interesting chapter on microcrystalline cellulose is described highlighting the importance of this widely used pharmaceutical excipient. Chapters related to recent advances in drug delivery systems are included to emphasize the latest trends in drug delivery systems. It includes a chapter dedicated to microbubbles for the management of AIDS. A chapter on pH-responsive microgels for controlled drug delivery is included highlighting the importance of stimuli-responsive drug delivery systems. Most of the current delivery systems are based on the passive approach, which means the drug struggles to reach the target site. Targeting various receptors inside the body not only enhances the pharmacological activity but also minimizes the toxicity and side effects associated with the drug. The brain has always been a challenge because of the presence of the blood brain barrier. The introduction of nanotechnology in pharmaceutical formulations has helped to successfully deliver and target the medication to treat various neurological disorders. A chapter describes the importance and approaches utilized in development of nanopharmaceuticals to target and treat brain disorders. A very interesting chapter on 3D printing of pharmaceuticals is described, which highlights the evolution and application of 3D printing technology in the healthcare sector.

This book aims to serve the need of all individuals involved at any level in the pharmaceutical dosage form development. I sincerely hope that the book will be liked by inquisitive students and learned colleagues.

Dr. Usama Ahmad
Assistant Professor,
Faculty of Pharmacy,
Integral University,
Lucknow, India

Section 1

Preformulation Study

Chapter 1

Preformulation Studies: An Integral Part of Formulation Design

Pinak Patel

Abstract

When a promising new chemical entity is synthesized, it needs transformation to appropriate formulation in order to show a better and desirable action at appropriate site. Preformulation study is a phase which is initiated once the new molecule is seeded. In a broader way, it deals with studies of physical, chemical, analytical, and pharmaceutical properties related to molecule and provides idea about suitable modification in molecule to show a better performance. Study of these parameters and suitable molecular modification can be linked to generation of effective, safer, stable, and reliable pharmaceutical formulation. Therefore, preformulation study is an approach for generation of pharmaceutical formulation which utilizes knowledge and area application of toxicology, biochemistry, medicinal chemistry, and analytical chemistry. The highlighted chapter is framed with a vision to provide an in-depth knowledge about pharmaceutical formulation development.

Keywords: preformulation, physicochemical properties, prodrug, stability studies, analytical profiling

1. Introduction

Discovery of a new drug entity is a huge milestone in science and it becomes even more important if it passes toxicity screening as the potential benefits overweigh the side effects. The ultimate effect of the new chemical entity depends on its availability at the site of action once it is administered through appropriate route in appropriate form. So for this reason, a new challenge is offered after successful pharmaceutical and toxicological screening that is to transform potential active new drug entity into a pharmaceutical formulation. It can be broadly elaborated as "a phase which works on study of physical, chemical, analytical, pharmacokinetic, and pharmacodynamic properties of new chemical entity and utilize the obtained results to design and develop an effective, stable, and a safer dosage form." Preformulation study is there for the multidisciplinary approach and utilizes involvement of several aspects of pharmacology, toxicology, clinical pharmacy, biochemistry, medicinal chemistry, and analytical chemistry (**Figure 1**). The preliminary objective of preformulation phase or study is to lay down foundation for transforming a new drug entity into a pharmaceutical formulation in such a way that it can be administered in a right way, in right amount, and on perhaps the most important at right target. The secondary objective preformulation study is to

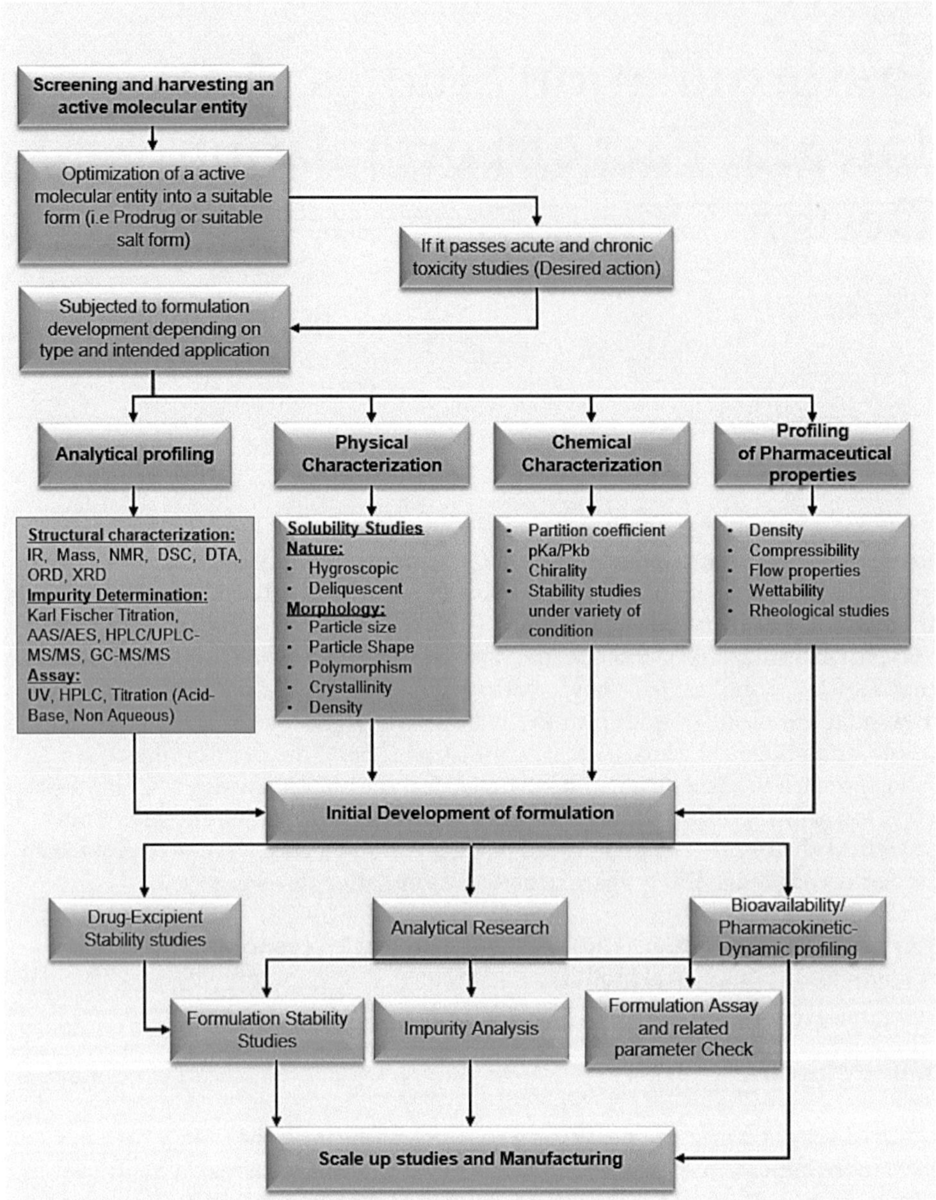

Figure 1.
Outline of preformulation studies.

provide longer stability to the formulation by proper designing and protecting drug component from environmental condition and to evaluate performance of developed formulation.

2. Optimization of an active molecular entity

Following the successful pharmacological screening of an active molecular entity, one has to be sure about the appropriate molecular form of active molecular entity. The optimization of molecule is needed with respect to stability of molecule under normal environmental condition or with respect to enhancing the performance of that molecule like bioavailability and stability. To inbuilt these virtues into a molecule, efforts are made to optimize a molecule inform of salts, solvates, polymorphs, and more importantly prodrug.

2.1 Salts

Nearly half of the drug molecules that are marketed as drug products are administered in salt form. Converting a molecule into a salt form is perhaps the most widely used approach to significantly enhance the performance of a molecule. This improvement can be made in area such as follows:

- Performance (increased solubility and bioavailability)
- Improved stability (hydrolytic and thermal stability)
- Better organoleptic properties (taste masking)
- Increased patient compliance (decreased side effects)
- Modified release dosage forms

There are several factors that are needed to be considered while selecting appropriate salt form. The main factor that determines the appropriate salt form is type of formulation that is to be developed.

- Mostly, sodium and hydrochloride are the most suitable forms to be used if formulation to be developed is tablet, oral solution, or injectable. With sodium and hydrochloride as salt form, there is always enhanced solubility and hence better bioavailability is assured. For example, the propionic acid derivative naproxen exists in free acid form and has lower water solubility and hence less bioavailability. When it is converted to sodium salt, its water solubility is increased by severalfold and hence better bioavailability is assured. Similarly, tolbutamide, an oral hypoglycemic agent has 1000-fold greater water solubility than corresponding free acidic form.

- Another factor that determines the type of salt form is type of formulation to be developed. For example, when the formulation to be developed is suspension, insoluble salt forms like tosylate, estylate, and embonate are the preferred salt forms.

- Therapeutic indication is another factor that affects the selection of salt form. For example, if drug is indicated in the treatment of hypertension, the use of sodium or potassium salt is avoided. This is the main reason behind development of potassium salt of diclofenac, which is preferred over sodium salt. Diclofenac potassium can be given as analgesic in patient with history or current occurrence of hypertension.

- As the regulatory perspective, selection of salt form must meet regulatory requirements and must be free from toxicity. For example, use of lithium salt is strictly prohibited.

- For immediate release formulations, generally sodium or hydrochloride salts are preferred as they show better solubility. For delayed release formulation, one can prefer low solubility salt form such as tosylate, estylate, and embonate.

- Increased patient compliance can be obtained by converting a molecule to a salt form. For instance, injection of cephalosporin generates the pain at site of application. However, when it is administered as morpholine salt, the pain at the site of application was reduced to many folds. In similar way, salt form can improve the taste adaptability by masking the taste and odor. Piperazine can be improved organolaptically by converting into salt with adipic acid [1].

2.2 Prodrug

Prodrug is the chemically modified inactive derivative of active form with optimized properties and better in vivo performance. Almost one-tenth of the pharmaceutical products are used as prodrug with main aim of improving bioavailability by avoiding first-pass metabolism, improved drug absorption, and organ selective transport. So prodrug can be defined as inactive form that undergoes biotransformation and converted to active form to elicit its pharmacological effect. Development of prodrug depends on specific property of drug that needs improvement and mostly with respect to stability, improving bioavailability [2].

In recent times, science has moved to "cod drugs," "hard drugs," and "soft drugs," where cod drug consists of two pharmacologically active components, which are complexed to form a single molecule (e.g., sulfasalazine, Levodopa-Entacapone). Soft drugs are the modified derivatives with predetermined metabolism, so that after exerting pharmacological action for suitable time, its metabolite can be eliminated from body. Main aim of developing soft drugs is to avoid toxicity associated with formed metabolites. Hard drugs are opposite to soft drugs, where the modifications are made in such a way that its original properties are retained but are not prone to chemical or biological transformation to avoid generation of metabolites or to increase the biological activity.

Apart from abovementioned classification, there are two main broad classes of prodrug that are carrier-linked prodrug and bioprecursor prodrug. In carrier-linked prodrug, the drug is linked to a carrier moiety by a temporary covalent linkage. Cleavage of a carrier prodrug generates a molecular entity of increased bioactivity (drug) and at least one side product, the carrier, which may be biologically inert. Carrier molecule or functional group can be easily removed in vivo, usually by hydrolytic cleavage [3]. There are several criteria for being a carrier-linked prodrug, which are as follows:

- Link between drug and a carrier molecule must be a covalent linkage.
- Carrier-linked prodrug is inactive or less active than the parent compound.
- The linkage between the drug and the carrier molecule must be broken in vivo.
- The prodrug, as well as the in vivo released transport moiety, must be nontoxic.
- The generation of the active form must take place with rapid kinetics to ensure effective drug levels at the site of action and to minimize either alternative prodrug metabolism or gradual drug inactivation.

Bioprecursor prodrug results from a molecular modification of the active principle. In vivo transformation of drug generates a new metabolite [4].

Several goals of developing prodrug are as follows:

Improving unfavorable physical properties:

- Improvement in water solubility.
- Improvement in lipophilicity.
- Improvement in chemical stability.
- Improvement in organoleptic characteristic.

Improving unfavorable pharmacokinetic properties:

- Improving bioavailability.
- Improving penetration power through membrane.
- Improved first-pass metabolism.
- Target-specific drug delivery.

Classical example of target-specific drug delivery in selective metastatic colon cancer is capecitabine which is prodrug of 5-fluorouracil. Capecitabine requires triple-phase transformation to be converted to its active form 5-fluorouracil. The first metabolism takes place in liver by action of enzyme carbonyl esterase. This transformed form then enters the tumor cells by selective uptake and is again transformed by deamination by action of enzyme cytidine deaminase. This form in tumor cell is converted to 5-fluorouracil by enzyme thymidine phosphorylase, which is only present in the tumor cells.

The other example of target-specific delivery is release of sulfasalazine in colon by action of bacterial reductase where sulfasalazine is converted to sulfapyridine and 5-amino salicylic, where the later formed is the active molecule.

One of the best ways to improve the lipophilicity is the esterification of the molecule. For example, terbutaline is orally active beta-2-agonist and is indicated in bronchial asthma. It requires significantly higher dose due to lower lipophilicity. Its prodrug bambuterol has improved lipophilicity as well as chemical stability and thus requires considerably lower dose than terbutaline [5].

3. Determination of chemical properties

Determination of chemical properties indicates the absorption behavior as well as stability of a molecule in the body. One of the most widely determined chemical properties includes partition coefficient (Log P), dissociation constant (pKa or pKb), and stability of molecule under a variety of conditions. Each property has significant value in development of formulation.

3.1 Partition coefficient

Partition coefficient (Log P) value is defined as ratio of unionized drug distributed between aqueous and organic phase. Oil-water partition coefficient gives the idea about drug's ability to cross the lipidic membrane. Lipophilic/hydrophilic balance is one of the most important contributing factors for optimum drug absorption and delivery. Due to lipidic nature of biological membrane, the amount of drug absorbed depends heavily on its lipophilicity. It is the unionized form of molecule that has better lipophilicity and hence it has received so much importance.

$$\text{Log P} = \left(\frac{\text{Coil}}{\text{Cwater}}\right)\text{equilibrium} \tag{1}$$

If the value of Log P is 0, it indicated that drug has equal distribution in water and partition solvent. Value of Log P less than 1 is indicative of higher water solubility and value greater than 1 is indicative of higher lipidic solubility. For optimum solubility and absorption, a proper hydrophilic-lipophilic balance is necessary.

Determination of Log P value in biological system is next to impossible task, so several methods are available to determine partition coefficient of molecule in vitro, which are as follows:

- Shake flask method
- Chromatographic method (HPLC)
- Computation based on software
- Countercurrent/filter probe method

Highly used method is shake flask method that utilizes octanol-water system to determine drug's partitioning behaviors. There are several reasons behind selection of octanol as partitioning solvent, which can be explained as follows:

- Octanol is believed to mimic the lipoidal character of biological membrane as it contains polar head and nonpolar tail.
- Octanol is organic compound that is immiscible with water; however, some of the water is expected to be present in polar head portion.
- Solubility parameter for most of the drugs resembles with that of octanol.

3.2 Dissociation constant

Like partition coefficient, dissociation constant (pKa) is the property that determines the solubility in pH-dependent environment and extent of ionization. It is the extent of ionization that determines the absorption as only unionized form can be absorbed and hence it becomes essential to determine the pKa value of molecule. pKa value determination gives idea about site of absorption.

Weakly acidic drugs having pKa value around 4 are best absorbed from stomach as they are predominantly present in unionized form. Basic drugs having pKa value of around 8 are best absorbed from intestine as they are predominantly present in unionized form. % ionization can be determined by the following equation:

$$\%\text{Ionization} = \left\{\frac{10^{(\text{pH}-\text{pKa})}}{1 + 10^{(\text{pH}-\text{pKa})}}\right\} \times 100 \tag{2}$$

Most of the strong acids and strong bases are present in ionized form throughout GIT and hence poorly absorbed. But it is also true that most of the pharmaceutical entities are derivatives of weak acids and weak bases and hence absorption is not an issue.

3.3 Chirality

One of the most silent chemical parameters that define the pharmacological activity is the type of isomer. Many molecular entities exist in racemic form, but only one form gives the desirable pharmacological activity. Other present isomer may be devoid of pharmacological activity or may exhibit deleterious side effects. Most of us are known to teratogenic tragedy of thalidomide. Thalidomide exists as racemic form. Racemates contain equal amount of enantiomer, which are known as either levorotatory (−) or dextrorotatory (+) based on its ability to rotate the plane of polarized light [6].

It was introduced as a sedative agent. The S-enantiomer of thalidomide was a teratogenic agent, while R-enantiomer was effective as a sedative agent. Lack of knowledge about chiral selectivity leads to disastrous consequence. In recent times, single enantiomer is dominating the market over the racemate form due to better pharmacological performance. Nowadays, racemic switching or chiral switching is used in which racemic mixtures are developed as single enantiomers. Several single enantiomers are preferred over racemic form (e.g., levofloxacin (ofloxacin), esomeprazole (omeprazole), escitalopram (citalopram), and desloratadine (loratadine)) [7].

Overview of the same is given in **Table 1**. For better clinical performance of the molecule, it has become necessity to study the chirality of the molecule. In most of the cases, it can be studied by optical rotatory dispersion and circular dichroism [8].

3.4 Stability of molecule

The main objective of determining stability of molecule is to identify the conditions in which molecule is susceptible to deteriorate and to determine degradation pathway. The mechanism of degradation and condition provides the idea about proper designing of formulation, suitable molecular modification, appropriate storage condition, and selection of proper packaging material.

Drug in racemic form	Used active enantiomer	Advantage offered
Ofloxacin	Levofloxacin S(−)-enantiomer	Enhanced activity against pneumococci
Cetirizine	Levocetirizine R(−)-enantiomer	Less sedative action with same activity
Ketoprofen	Dexketoprofen S(+)-enantiomer	Reduction is dose of ketoprofen (half) with same effectiveness and lesser GT-related side effects
Ibuprofen	S(+)-enantiomer	(S)-ibuprofen is over 100-fold more potent inhibitor of cyclooxygenase. So three times dose reduction was achieved than racemic mixture
Omeprazole	Esomeprazole S(+)-enantiomer	Esomeprazole has lower first-pass metabolism and shows better bioavailability than R-eneantiomer and maintains pH above 4 in patients with GERD with least variability
Salbutamol	Levalbuterol	Racemic for and S-enantiomer hyperresponsiveness in sensitized patients with loss of bronchodilator activity. (*R*)-salbutamol produces significantly greater bronchodilation than the equivalent dose of the racemate

Table 1.
Advantage of racemic switching.

The major mechanisms by which a molecule undergoes degradation are hydrolysis, oxidation, photolysis, and racemization. Out of these mechanisms, hydrolysis is perhaps the most studied after oxidation.

3.4.1 Hydrolysis

Hydrolysis involves reaction of a molecule with water resulting in cleavage of a chemical bond within the molecule. If readily hydrolyzable functional groups are available, then reaction proceeds even at faster rates, making the molecule ineffective. Molecules containing esters and amide functional groups are prone to hydrolysis and especially the ester derivatives, which may lead to formation of carboxylic acid or an alcohol.

- Effectiveness of molecule therefore depends on hydrolytic stability of molecule. For example, lidocaine is amide derivative of procaine, which is ester derivative used as local anesthetic. As ester derivative is more readily hydrolyzed; its duration of action is short while amide derivative is more stable and hence used as long-acting local anesthetic.

- Beta-lactam antibiotics are susceptible to hydrolysis and hence they are supplied as dry powder injection where they are reconstituted before intravenous administration.

3.4.2 Oxidation

Many molecules can undergo oxidative degradation, which involves exposure of molecule to atmospheric oxygen or autoxidation by free radicals. However, in some cases, oxidation can be initiated in presence of light or elevated temperature. So degree of oxidation can be controlled by avoiding exposure to lights and storage at controlled temperatures. Even the extent of oxidation can be controlled by addition of antioxidants. The extent of oxidation for a given substance can be studied by passing oxygen through the solution of substance, or it can be achieved by addition of hydrogen peroxide to the solution of substance.

3.4.3 Photolysis

Photolysis refers to decomposition of a molecule by absorption of energy when exposed to light. Exposure to light not only brings photodegradation but may trigger oxidation. It is absorption of shorter wavelength components that may bring oxidation than longer wavelength components. Prior knowledge of photochemical behavior can provide guidance regarding storage condition, packaging, and handling condition. In most of the cases, the photochemical behavior of molecule is studied in the range of different spectral regions that are 200–290, 290–320, 320–400, and 400–700 nm. For example, riboflavin and vitamin B12 are susceptible to photodegradation directly and oxidation induced by light. So to avoid the decomposition, the formulation containing vitamin B12 and riboflavin is stored in amber color vials. Amber color bottles do not allow the ultraviolet radiation to pass through, which is the main factor for photodegradation [9].

3.4.4 Racemization

It is an event where optically active molecule becomes inactive without any change in molecular composition. Such study is of highest importance when racemic mixture form is used. Racemization leads to either loss of pharmacological action or toxic effect may be enhanced by severalfold. Racemization is mostly affected by the conditions like pH, type of solvents, presence of light, and temperature. So main goal in this study is to design optimum condition in which molecule can remain stable [10].

4. Physical characterization of molecule

Most often than not, new chemical entity exists in solid form and the properties under study during preformulation phase are bulk property characterization and micromeritic property characterization. Bulk property characterization includes study of polymorphism, crystallinity, density, nature of molecule like deliquescence or hygroscopicity and micromeritic characterization includes study of particle size, shape, porosity, and density. As most of the new chemical entities are solids, they exist either as amorphous or in crystalline state. Either of the form imparts the two main virtues that are stability and solubility.

4.1 Solubility

One of the most widely studied techniques during preformulation analysis is solubility profile of drug candidate. It is the backbone study of preformulation stage that determines the performance of developed formulation. Solubility and permeability forms the scientific basis of biopharmaceutics classification system (BCS), which can provide framework for designing type of drug delivery system. **Table 2** provides basic idea about basic BCS classification and link between solubility, permeability, and type of targeted formulation.

The solubility of a drug is the amount of the drug that dissolves in a given solvent to produce a saturated solution at constant temperature and pressure. **Table 3** provides outline of different levels of solubility. For conversion of drug molecule into an effective oral formulation, it must have good aqueous solubility for better absorption. Solubility is not an independent parameter but it relies on several properties like crystal characteristics, temperature, pH, complexation, and molecular structure. There are several techniques, which are available to improve the solubility of drug candidate, which are as follows:

- Chemical modification of drug
- Addition of cosolvent or surfactant
- Particle size reduction
- Hydrotropy
- Complexation

4.2 Crystalline vs amorphous form

Amorphous drugs have randomly arranged molecules or atoms in the molecular lattice. Typical amorphous forms are obtained by techniques like precipitation, rapid cooling after melting, and lyophilization. One of the most important advantages associated with amorphous form is the higher solubility and hence the higher dissolution rate. More often than not drugs with low water solubility lead to poor bioavailability and variable clinical response. So, polymorphic form may overcome this problem

BCS class	Solubility	Permeability	Approaches in formulation development
Class 1	High	High	Conventional solid oral dosage form
Class 2	Low	High	Use techniques to improve surface area or improving solubility by addition of cosolvents or surfactants
Class 3	High	Low	Use of permeability enhances
Class 4	Low	Low	Use approaches of classes 2 and 3

Table 2.
Correlation of solubility and permeability with BCS class and associated approach in formulation development.

Descriptive term	Part of solvent required for one part of solute
Very soluble	Less than 1
Freely soluble	1–10
Soluble	10–30
Sparingly soluble	30–100
Slightly soluble	100–1000
Very slightly soluble	1000–10,000
Practically insoluble or insoluble	10,000 or more

Table 3.
Solubility description.

with main challenge of stability. The associated disadvantage is the reduced stability in comparison to crystalline form, so upon storage, amorphous forms tend to revert to more stable form. But the risk-to-benefit ratio remains in the favor of amorphous from and hence is more preferred for product development. For example, novobiocin when administered in crystalline form showed no therapeutic activity, while amorphous from showed better absorption from gastrointestinal tract with significant therapeutic response [11]. Crystalline form is characterized by regular spacing between molecular lattices in three-dimensional structure. One of the striking advantages associated with this form is the impeccable stability at a cost of lower water solubility than amorphous form. For example, Penicillin G as sodium or potassium salt in crystalline form has the better stability and hence stable and better therapeutic response in comparison to amorphous form. Various techniques are available to study crystallinity like X-ray, differential scanning microscopy, differential thermal analysis, hot stage microscopy, and the most important one that is scanning electron microscopy.

4.3 Polymorphism and pseudo polymorphism

Polymorphism is the ability of a compound to crystallize as more than one distinct chemically identical crystalline species with different internal lattices or crystal packing arrangement. Type of crystalline species generated depends on temperature, solvent, and time. Polymorphs are chemically same but mainly differ with respect to physical and pharmaceutical properties. As different types of polymorphs exhibit different types of solubility, stability, and therapeutic activity, it has become mandatory to have preliminary and exhaustive screening to identify all the polymorphic crystal forms for each drug. Similarly, chloramphenicol palmitate exists in three different polymorphic forms, namely, A, B, and C. Form

B has higher solubility and better dissolution profile, while form A is more stable one but low serum concentration was observed. During formulating suspension of an anthelmintic drug oxyclozanide, transformation of unstable polymorph to more stable leads to different crystal size and causes caking. In case of creams, crystal growth leads to gritty texture and incase of suppositories one can observe different melting behaviors and leads to formulation instability [12]. When solvent molecules are incorporated into structure of drug molecule, it is known as solvate. When water is incorporated as solvent in the structure, they are termed as hydrates. Pseudopolymorphs are the different crystal form of solvates. This phenomenon is also referred to as solvomorphism. For example, during synthesis of ethinylestradiol, crystallization of final product is achieved by using solvents like acetonitrile, chloroform, methanol, and water. As a result, four different solvates are generated. Differentiation of pseudopolymorphs can be studied by hot stage microscopy (melting behavior). True polymorphs melt slightly and form a globule, while pseudopolymorphs give bubble in the system due to generation of vapor or gas from entrapped solvent.

Two different types of polymorphs are well defined and are known as "monotropic polymorphs" and "enantiotropic polymorphs." Monotropic polymorph can be reversibly changed into another form by change in temperature and pressure and the latter involves one-time transition into another form. With respect to stability and solubility, again polymorphs can be classified as stable and metastable polymorphs. Stable polymorph is one of the most physically stable polymorphic forms and has highest melting point, lowest energy, and least aqueous solubility, while metastable polymorph refers to forms other than stable polymorph and has highest energy, low melting point, highest aqueous solubility, and hence shows better bioavailability. Metastable polymorphs have wider application in developing formulation but still only one-tenth of metastable forms are having practical use as they suffer from the stability issues [13].

4.4 Deliquescency vs hygroscopicity

Hygroscopicity can be defined as the capacity of a compound to absorb atmospheric moisture. Amount of moisture absorbed depends on atmospheric conditions and surface area. Deliquescent substance absorbs moisture to a greater extent and liquefies itself. The main reason behind study of this property is because changes in the moisture level can influence chemical stability, flowability, and compressibility to a greater extent.

In European pharmacopeia, hygroscopicity is described by four different classes after being stored at 25°C at relative humidity of 80% for 24 hours.

- Slightly hygroscopic: After abovementioned storage condition, if overall increase in weight is greater or equal to 0.2% but less than 2% w/w.

- Hygroscopic: After abovementioned storage condition, if overall increase in weight is greater or equal to 0.2% but less than 15% w/w.

- Very hygroscopic: After abovementioned storage condition, if overall increase in weight is greater than 15% w/w.

For this study, samples under analysis are exposed to range of controlled relative humidity prepared with saturated aqueous salt solutions (**Table 4**). One can link flowability and relative humidity by amount of moisture uptake (**Table 5**).

Moisture level uptake can be monitored by techniques like thermogravimetric analysis (TGA), Karl Fischer titration, and gas chromatography.

Substance used	% RH achieved
Silica gel	0%
Potassium acetate	20%
Calcium chloride	30%
Potassium bromide	85%
Water	100%

Table 4.
Utilization of different salts to give environment with different RH.

Process	Affected properties
Precipitation	Surface area, particle size, shape
Encapsulation	Particle shape and size
Crystallization	Particle shape, size, crystalline/amorphous nature
Chemical reaction	Surface area and particle shape

Table 5.
Use of different process to control particle size, shape, and surface area.

4.5 Particle size

Particle size greatly affects a number of quality parameters like dissolution rate, solubility, bioavailability, content uniformity, and lack of grittiness. Application of particle size study during preformulation stage is described as follows:

- When solubility is major issue, one may significantly improve the solubility by reducing the particle size (increased surface area).
- In case of suspension, particle size is the most important parameter, which determines the stability and quality of formulation. Too much reduction in the particle size leads to generation of charged particle and hence unstable system. On other hand, larger particle size leads to caking.
- Due to nonuniform particle size distribution, there is significant risk associated with content uniformity in case of potent formulations.

A number of methods are available to determine particle size, which are as follows:

- Microscopy
- Sedimentation rate
- Coulter counter method
- Surface area determination by nitrogen adsorption method

Apart from particle size, particle shape plays an important role during preformulation phase as the shape of particle may influence surface area, flow properties, and compaction force. A drug particle may exist in different forms like spherical, angular, acicular, needle, oval, or rough. It is a well-accepted fact that a spherical particle has the maximum area and uniform flow property. The maximum surface area ensures the better solubility. For topical products that are working as abrasives, irregular particle shape is more preferred. **Table 3** provides idea about various methods, which can control particle shape and size and provide better results needed to design a formulation.

4.6 Density and porosity

Density can be defined as ratio of mass of a substance to its volume, which greatly depends on particle size distribution and shape. The main problem arises during determination of bulk volume is the voids, which can be interparticulate, open, and closed intraparticulate. So by considering the presence of different types of void volume, various densities are proposed.

- True density: It is defined as total volume of solids excluding all space greater than molecule diameter. True density can be measured with helium pycnometer.

- Bulk density: It is defined as total volume occupied by entire powder mass. It can be determined by placing previously sieved powder bulk into a graduated cylinder and measuring the volume in milliliters. Division of original weight and attended volume gives idea about bulk density.

- Tapped density: It is determined by placing graduated cylinder containing known weight of sample on tapped density apparatus and is operated for the fixed number of taps until a constant volume is attained. Ratio of total amount of substance taken to the final constant volume gives idea about tapped density.

One needs to gain knowledge about the size and type of dosage form and is the most critical parameter for the low potency drugs. In most of the cases, two types of density are studied, namely, bulk density and tapped density.

Following problems can be addressed related to density:

- With drugs having low density, the bulk becomes more and hence capsule formulation is quite difficult to formulate as capsule can incorporate limited volume.

- In development of tablet formulation, low-density drug creates difficulties as they are having low compressibility and hardness in tablet is difficult to achieve.

- If the difference of density is more between drug substances and excipient is more, homogeneity in the formulation is difficult to achieve.

4.7 Flow properties

Flow property of material can be affected by a number of factors including frictional forces, surface tension forces, electric forces, and van der Waals forces.

Efficient flow of drug substance powder is needed for effective tablet formulation. The main reason behind inclusion of this parameter in preformulation is its linkage with other physical parameters like hygroscopicity and particle size and shape. Importance of flow property is even more when dose loading is more.

Table 6 gives outline on correlation of flow properties of a material with moisture uptake at different humidity levels.

- In case of hygroscopic material, flow property of drug tends to deteriorate as the presence of absorbed moisture increases cohesiveness.
- Irregular particle size and nonuniform shape can also disturb normal flow property of drug.

Normally, flow property of solid drug substance can be measured by Hausner ratio, Carr's index, and angle of repose, and in case of liquids or semisolid, rheology and thixotropy. Carr's compressibility index can be represented by the following formula.

$$\text{Carr's compressibility index} = \frac{\text{Tapped density} - \text{Bulk density}}{\text{Tapped density}} \times 100. \quad (3)$$

Hausner's ratio can be represented by the following equation:

$$\text{Hausner's ratio} = \frac{\text{Tapped density}}{\text{Bulk density}}. \quad (4)$$

Table 7 provides the correlation between Carr's index, Hausner's ratio, and flowability.

Another way of measuring flow property is angle of repose, which provides the idea resistance to the movement of particle. It can be represented by the following formula:

$$\tan\theta = 2h/D \quad (5)$$

Relative humidity (%)	Moisture uptake (%)	Flowability
1	0.30	Free flowing
10	0.24	Free flowing
20	0.27	Less free flowing
40	0.35	Base of powder adheres to the container
80	0.62	Cake formation

Table 6.
Correlation between relative humidity, moisture uptake, and flowability.

Carr's index	Hausner's ratio	Flowability
5–15	1.05–1.18	Excellent
12–16	1.14–1.20	Good
18–21	1.22–1.26	Fair-passable
23–35	1.30–1.54	Poor
33–38	1.50–1.61	Very poor
Greater than 40	Greater than 1.67	Very very poor

Table 7.
Correlation between Carr's index, Hausner's ration, and flowability.

It is the maximum angle that can be obtained between height of pile and a horizontal plane. It gives a brief idea about internal cohesive and frictional levels. There are basically two types of methods that are available, which are as follows:

Static angle of repose

1. Fixed funnel method

2. Fixed cone method

Dynamic angle of repose

1. Rotating cylinder method

2. Tilting box method

5. Drug excipient compatibility

Excipients are added along with the active pharmaceutical ingredient in formulations. Most excipients possess biological activity but having role in administration, mediating the release of the active component, and providing stability against degradation. However, inappropriate excipients can also give rise to inadvertent and/or unintended effects, which can affect the chemical nature, the stability, and the bioavailability of the API, and consequently, their therapeutic efficacy and safety. So study about interaction between active ingredient and inactive ingredient can provide idea about type of incompatibility and the justification behind the inactive ingredient selection [14].

- Change in organoleptic properties of formulation.

- Changes in in vivo performance of formulation, that is, dissolution.

- Decreased potency of active ingredient.

- Generation of toxic degradation product.

- Change in physical appearance of formulation, that is, color, phase conversion.

In general, one can say that drug-excipient incompatibility may result in change in physical, chemical, microbiological, or therapeutic properties of formulation.

5.1 Physical incompatibility

In such an instance, active pharmaceutical ingredient and excipients interact without undergoing changes involving like breaking or formation of new bonds. The resulting drug product retains its original chemical properties but may involve changes such as alteration in physical properties. Such interaction results in changes like change in color, odor, flow properties, and sedimentation rate. Such an example of physical incompatibility is between tetracycline and calcium carbonate. It results in formation of insoluble complex with calcium carbonate, leading to slower dissolution and decreased absorption in the gastrointestinal tract [15].

5.2 Chemical incompatibility

In such incompatibility, there is interaction of active pharmaceutical ingredient and excipient through chemical degradation pathway. The chemical reaction involves bond breakage or new bond formation to produce an unstable chemical entity. Chemical reaction may take place as hydrolysis, oxidation racemization, and Maillard reactions. The resulting changes are more deleterious than physical incompatibility. This type of incompatibility can be assessed by chromatographic studies. One of the classical examples of chemical incompatibility is exhibited by reaction of lactose with amino group of active pharmaceutical ingredient referred to as "Maillard reaction" and results into darkening of formulation with characteristic odor. Classical example is of a bronchodilator aminophylline, in which ethylenediamine moiety is reduced by lactose and as a result brown discoloration appeared in samples containing 1:5 (w/w) mixtures of aminophylline and lactose after storing at 60°C for 3 weeks [16].

5.3 Therapeutic incompatibility

Such interaction is also referred to as biopharmaceutical interaction, but it differs from previously discussed incompatibilities in a way that interaction will take place once the formulation is administered into the body. Such type of incompatibility is associated with alteration in drug absorption in the body. In other way, one can say that interaction is taking place between excipient, active component, and physiological fluid. One of the classical examples of such incompatibility is interaction of enteric coated polymers, when administered along with antacids. In such an event, they dissolve prematurely and release the drug that is liable to acid degradation or may cause adverse effect in GI, that is, gastric bleeding associated with NSAIDs [17].

There are specific methods that are employed to determine the existence of incompatibility between excipient and the active pharmaceutical ingredient. Out of all analytical techniques, thermal methods of analysis can provide most positive outcome. In association with thermal methods of analysis, spectroscopic techniques like X-ray diffraction and infrared spectroscopy can provide sideline assistance. High-performance liquid chromatography and thin-layer chromatography provide the more suitable way of studying chemical incompatibilities and provide qualitative and quantitative assessments.

6. Conclusion

It can be concluded that preformulation is a proactive phase that deals with transformation of new chemical entity into a safe, effective, and most importantly stable pharmaceutical formulation.

Author details

Pinak Patel
Smt. S.M. Shah Pharmacy College, Mehemdabad, India

*Address all correspondence to: pinakqa@gmail.com

References

[1] Sigfridsson K, Nilsson L, Ahlqvist M, Andersson T, Granath AK. Preformulation investigation and challenges; salt formation, salt disproportionation and hepatic recirculation. European Journal of Pharmaceutical Sciences. 2017;**104**: 262-272. DOI: 10.1016/j.ejps.2017.03.041

[2] Abet V, Filace F, Recio J, Builla JA, Burgos C. Prodrug approach: An overview of recent cases. European Journal of Medicinal Chemistry. 2017;**127**:810-827. DOI: 10.1016/j.ejmech.2016.10.061

[3] Lohar V, Singhal S, Arora V. Prodrug: Approach to better drug delivery. International Journal of Pharmaceutical Research. 2012;**4**(1):15-21

[4] Hajnal K, Gabriel H, Aura R, Erzsébet V, Blanka SS. Prodrug strategy in drug development. Acta Medica Marisiensis. 2016;**62**(3):356-362. DOI: 10.1515/amma-2016-0032

[5] Bhosle D, Bharambe S, Gairola N, et al. Mutual prodrug concept: Fundamentals and applications. International Journal of Pharmaceutical Research. 2006;**68**(3):286-294

[6] Chabra N, Aseri ML, Padmanabhan D. A Review on Drug Isomerism and its Significance. International Journal of Applied Basic Medical Research. 2013;**3**(1):16-18. DOI: 10.4103/2229-516X.112233

[7] Smith SW. Chiral toxicology: It's the same thing...only different. Toxicological Sciences. 2009;**110**(1): 4-30. DOI: 10.1093/toxsci/kfp097

[8] Black K, Raissy H. Chiral switch drugs for asthma and allergies: True benefit or marketing hype. Pediatric Allergy, Immunology, and Pulmonology. 2013;**26**(3):157-160. DOI: 10.1089/ped.2013.0285

[9] Gohel MC. Overview on chirality and applications of stereo-selective dissolution testing in the formulation and development work. Dissolution Technologies. 2003;**10**(3):16-20. DOI: 10.14227DT100303P16

[10] Iqbal A, Sofia A, Zubair A, Ali SM, Sikorski M. Photo stability and photo stabilization of drugs and drug products. International Journal of Photoenergy. 2016:1-19. DOI: 10.1155/2016/8135608

[11] Babak J, Inga B, Ole N, Steen HH. Investigation of racemization of the enantiomers of glitazone drug compounds at different pH using chiral HPLC and chiral CE. Journal of Pharmaceutical and Biomedical Analysis. 2008;**46**(1):82-87. DOI: 10.1016/j.jpba.2007.09.004

[12] Censi R, Di Martino P. Polymorph impact on the bioavailability and stability of poorly soluble drugs. Molecules. 2015;**20**:18759-18776. DOI: 10.3390/molecules201018759

[13] Chaurasia G. A review on pharmaceutical preformulation studies in formulation and development of new drug molecules. International Journal of Pharmaceutical Sciences and Research. 2016;**7**(6):2313-2320. DOI: 10.13040/IJPSR.0975-8232.7(6).2313-20

[14] Verma G, Mishra M. Pharmaceutical Preformulation studies in formulation and development of new dosage form: A review. International Journal of Pharma Research & Review. 2016;**5**(10):12-20

[15] Patel P, Ahir K, Patel V, Patel C. Drug-excipient compatibility studies: First step for dosage form development. The Pharma Innovation Journal. 2015;**4**(5):14-20

[16] Bharate SS, Bharate SB, Bajaj AN. Interactions and incompatibilities

of pharmaceutical excipients with active pharmaceutical ingredients: A comprehensive review. Journal of Excipients and Food Chemicals. 2010;**1**(3):3-26

[17] Shadbad MR, Ghaderi F, Hatami L. Investigation of possible Maillard reaction between acyclovir and dextrose upon dilution prior to parenteral administration. AAPS PharmSciTech. 2016;**17**(6):1491-1499. DOI: 10.1208/s12249-016-0494-2

Chapter 2

Drug Analysis

Shaza W. Shantier

Abstract

Instrumental methods are widely used for the analysis and stability studies of compounds in bulk and pharmaceutical forms. They vary in their sensitivity, techniques and reagents involved. This chapter will overview those different techniques and the application of the analytical methods. It will also describe how to design and develop simple, sensitive and accurate method for routine quality control of specified compound depending on its molecular structure. Quality control and assurance of the analytical process will be discussed. Furthermore, the chapter will describe a number of factors affecting the chemical and physical stability of Pharmaceutical formulations and how to develop stability-indicating methods to qualify and quantify the drug degradation.

Keywords: instrumental, development, quality control, validation, stability

1. Introduction

Drug discovery and development process can be divided into two major stages: drug discovery which involves isolation of the active constituent, purified, and standardized. The second major stage, drug development, starts with a solitary compound, which at that point progresses through different studies intended to support its endorsement as a new drug [1]. The new drug will then be formulated as an appropriate pharmaceutical dosage form.

Pharmaceutical product is medicine intended for human or veterinary use in cure, alleviation, prevention or diagnosis of disease. The use of ineffective, harmful or poor-quality drugs will cause health hazards and waste of funds. The problem is aggravated by adverse climatic conditions and weak drug supply system (including storage and transport). These lead to deterioration of drug quality, loss of activity and may be formation of harmful degradation products [2]. All this made it a must that any pharmaceutical product should be subjected to different analytical procedures in order to ensure its efficacy and safety. Therefore, an effective drug quality assurance and assessment system should be developed and maintained.

2. Pharmaceutical analysis

Broadly speaking, this is the application of a process in order to identify a drug (single or combined) in its bulk or pharmaceutical dosage form. Testing pharmaceutical product involves chemical, physical and sometimes microbiological analysis [3].

Pharmaceutical analysis can be divided into two types of methods:

a. Qualitative methods: these methods usually are used to ascertain the presence or identity of a component and\or impurities (predicted or expected).

b. Quantitative methods: determine how much of known drugs are present in bulk form or in a formulation.

Since the judgment for quality of a drug depends on the method of analysis used, the validity or control of the method used is required. The methods used in pharmaceutical analysis should be capable of:

a. Correct identification of the drug in bulk form or as a formulated product.

b. Indicating the percentage of the stated content of a drug present in formulation within acceptable stated limits.

c. Indicating the stability of the drug in the formulation and hence the shelf life i.e. indicating the presence of a drug in its intact form and or the presence of any impurities (whether as drug precursors, decomposition products due to chemical or photochemical causes).

d. Application in the dissolution rate studies i.e. at what rate is the drug released from its formulation so that can be absorbed by the body (bioavailability studies).

e. Ensuring that the identity and purity of pure drug (bulk form) meet official standards or monograph.

f. Ensuring that the identity and purity of excipients used in formulation meet specifications set by official standards.

g. Indicating the concentration of the specified impurities in the pure drug substance (limit test application).

3. Drug stability

The stability of a pharmaceutical product is defined as the capability of the product, in a specific container, to retain its efficacy, properties and characteristics throughout its shelf-life [4]. The recommended shelf-life (expiry date) for a commercial pharmaceutical product is 3–5 years. During this time, the concentration of the drug should not be reduced more than 95% of its value when originally prepared [5].

There are five types of stability that concern the pharmacist in the manufacturing of drugs:

a. Chemical (including photochemical): the product retains its chemical integrity and potency.

b. Physical: the conformity of the pharmaceutical product (color, appearance, dissolution, etc.) does not change upon storage or handling.

c. Microbiological: sterilized products should remain sterile (no pyrogenicity).

d. Therapeutic: the therapeutic effect remains unchanged within the specified dosage regimen.

e. Toxicological: no significant increase in a predetermined toxicity effect is noted.

Stability types (therapeutic, microbiological, and toxicological) are basically dependent on the chemical and physical properties of the drug.

Knowledge of the chemical stability of a drug is of great concern for selecting suitable storage condition against the effects of light, temperature, humidity, etc. and for anticipation of drugs interaction with each other or with excipients [6, 7].

A stable drug is of great concern to the pharmacist (in view of marketing, storage and distribution); to the physician and patient (in view of safety and efficacy); and to the regulator and quality control analyst (in view of quality, strength, purity and identity).

3.1 Chemical reactions that cause drug degradation

Many drugs are derivatives of carboxylic acid or contain functional groups based on this moiety, for example esters, amides, lactones, lactams, imides or carbamates [5]. Accordingly, various chemical reactions can result in the degradation of the drug. These reactions include hydrolysis, oxidation, photochemical reactions, polymerization, isomerization, racemization and dehydration [4, 5, 8].

3.1.1 Hydrolysis (or solvolysis)

Hydrolysis forms the most common pathway by which drugs become degraded since many drugs contain hydrolysable functional groups. It can be defined as the process by which drug molecules interact with water to yield breakdown products of different chemical constitution. Hydrolysis occurs more readily in liquid state than in the solid state. It may occur in aqueous suspensions of sparingly soluble drugs. In tablets and other solid dosage forms, there may be sufficient water to allow hydrolysis of the drug [8].

Solvolysis is a term used for the reactions involving the decomposition of the active drugs with their solvent present (not water).

3.1.2 Ester hydrolysis

Hydrolysis of drugs with an ester functional group (e.g. procaine, atropine, etc.) forms one of the most common types of drug instability. It is usually a bimolecular reaction involving acyl-oxygen cleavage. Ester hydrolysis is (H^+) or (OH^-) ion catalyzed and is dependent on the specific compound and the pH of the solution. Atropine hydrolysis is totally pH dependent and this was characterized by the slopes of −1 and +1. In some cases, the hydrolysis of the drug can show a pH-profile with three regions: a hydrogen ion (proton) catalyzed region, (slope = −1), an uncatalyzed region (solvent dependent, slope = 0) and a hydroxyl ion-catalyzed region (slope = +1) (**Figure 1**) [5].

3.1.3 Amide hydrolysis

Amides are generally more stable to hydrolysis than esters. In general the rate of hydroxyl ion-catalyzed reaction of amides is greater than the proton-catalyzed hydrolysis [6].

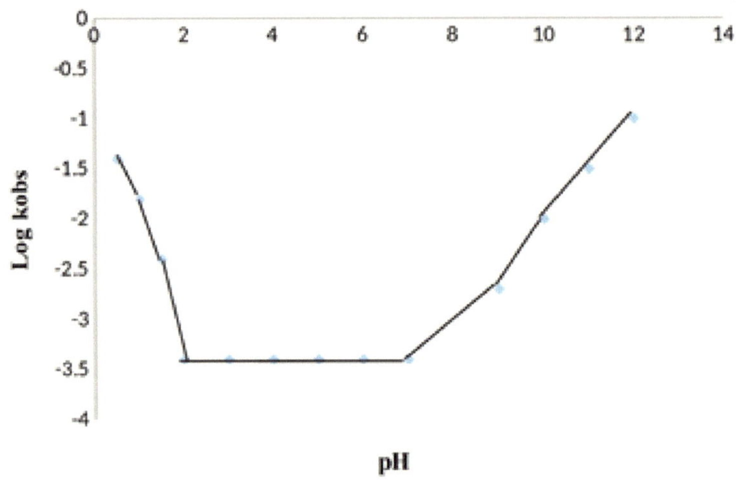

Figure 1.
Log rate-pH profile for the degradation of atropine at 60°C.

Penicillins and cephalosporins are amides in which the amide bond is part of the strained four membered ß-lactam rings. Their decomposition is catalyzed by hydrogen ion, hydroxyl ion and many buffers. Therefore, these compounds are too unstable to be formulated as solutions. Their pH profile is generally similar to the pH-profile shown in **Figure 1**.

In addition to acid-base catalyzed hydrolysis, enzyme-catalyzed hydrolysis may take place in drugs of natural origin; for example enzymes catalyzes the hydrolysis of cardiac glycosides in digitalis leaf [8].

3.1.4 Oxidation

Oxidation involves the removal of an electropositive atom, radical or electron, or the addition of an electronegative atom or radical. When a reaction involves molecular oxygen (O—O), it is commonly called autoxidation and this forms the most common pathway of oxidative decomposition of pharmaceuticals.

Oxidative degradation by autoxidation may involve chain processes consisting of three concurrent reactions—initiation, propagation and termination. Initiation can be via free radicals formed from organic compounds by the action of light, heat or transition metals such as copper and iron which are present in trace amounts in almost every buffer [5].

Many drugs are complex molecules and can be subjected to both hydrolysis and oxidation e.g. steroids, anti-inflammatory, polyene antibiotics (amphotericin B) etc.

Figure 2 show the oxidation of phenothiazines to the sulfoxide which involves two single-electron transfer reactions involving a radical cation intermediate. The sulfoxide is subsequently formed by reaction of the cation with water [5].

Oxidation in solution generally follows first or second order kinetics. Some oxidation reactions are redox reactions that involve the loss of electrons without the addition of oxygen e.g. oxidation of ascorbic acid, ferrous sulfate, adrenaline and riboflavin [8].

In addition to oxidation and hydrolysis, many other degradative reactions had been studied including addition, dehydration, polymerization, isomerization, acylation, transesterification, etc.

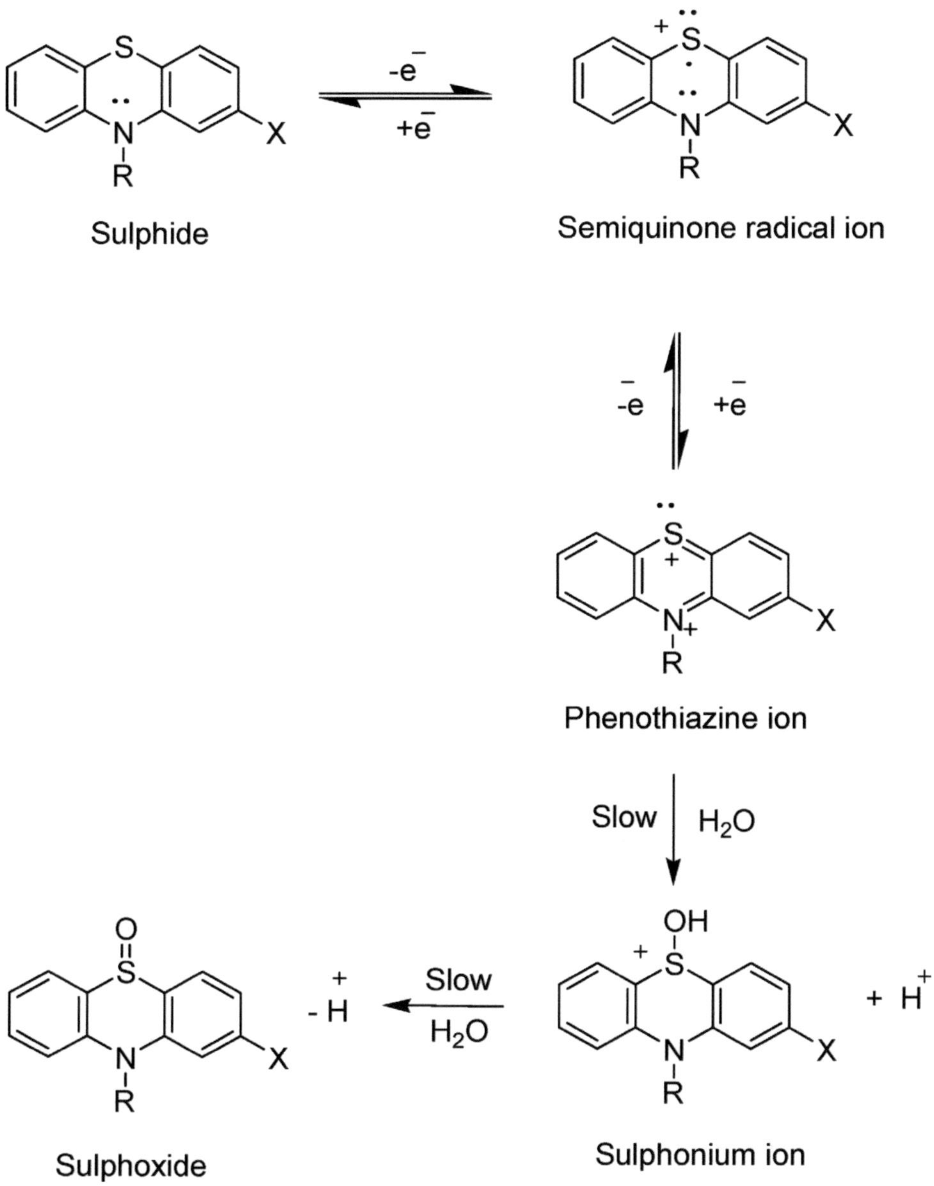

Figure 2.
Phenothiazine oxidation process.

3.1.5 Photochemical degradation

These are the reactions that take place by absorption of the visible or ultraviolet light. The reactant molecule absorbs photons of light (energy) and get excited. The excited molecule then produces the photodecomposition product.

In many photochemical reactions, the reactant molecule may not absorb the radiation directly but through a mediator which absorbs the incident radiation and subsequently transfers its energy to the reactant molecule that becomes activated. Such type of mediator is called photosensitizer.

At times, a molecule can act as a protector for the photolabile drug by preferentially absorbing the radiant energy and produce products. These compounds are referred to as screening agents [9].

3.1.5.1 Light sources for photodegradation studies

The majority of therapeutic substances are white in appearance, which means that they may absorb in the UV region depending on their chemical structure.

Grossweiner, 1989 [10], divided the ultraviolet radiation (UV-R) into three sub-bands:

1. UV-C: which ranges between 200 and 290 nm and is termed shortwave or far UV. Sunlight at the earth's surface is devoid of this band due to its absorption by molecular oxygen and ozone in the upper atmosphere. Artificial radiation sources such as discharge and germicidal lamps and welding arcs form the sources of UV-C which are used for forced drug photodegradation studies (stress-conditions). These also cause serious damage to the skin and cornea [11].

2. UV-B band: this covers the region 280–320 nm. It causes sunburn, skin cancer and other biological effects and it is responsible for the direct photoreaction of many chemicals in natural sunlight.

3. UV-A band: this is the long wavelength region from 320 to 400 nm, also called near-UV because it is near the visible region.

The most commonly sources for photostability studies include: day light, window-glass filtered day light and room light [12]. All these sources can be generated artificially. The artificial light source should have an output with spectral power distribution (SPD) as near as possible to the sunlight. This can be achieved by the use of arc lamps and fluorescent tubes.

3.1.5.2 Drug molecules labile to photodecomposition

A number of medicinal products have been studied for their photostability. Carbonyl, nitroaromatic and *N*-oxide functions, aryl halides, alkenes, polyenes and sulfides are certain chemical functions that are expected to introduce photoreactivity [13].

Photodegradation of a drug is considered of practical significance if the compound absorbs light >300 nm and the photodegradation becomes evident in a short period.

Factors that govern photochemical reaction rate include aerobic (most reactions proceed in presence of oxygen) and anaerobic (N_2) conditions, solvents (H_2O, organic solvents), buffers, temperature, metals, intensity of radiation and spectral distribution of light, drug concentration and volume of the sample [14].

Thus, in formulations that contain low drug concentrations, the primary photochemical reaction follows first-order kinetics; the kinetics is more complicated at higher concentrations and in the solid state because most of the light is then absorbed near the surface of the product.

The mechanisms of photodegradation are of such complexity as to have been fully elucidated in only a few cases. For example, the phenothiazine chlorpromazine (CLP) is rapidly decomposed under the action of ultraviolet light, the decomposition being accompanied by discoloration of the solutions (**Figure 3**). Chlorpromazine behaves differently towards ultraviolet irradiation under anaerobic conditions.

A polymerization process has been proposed which involves the liberation of HCl in its initial stages [5].

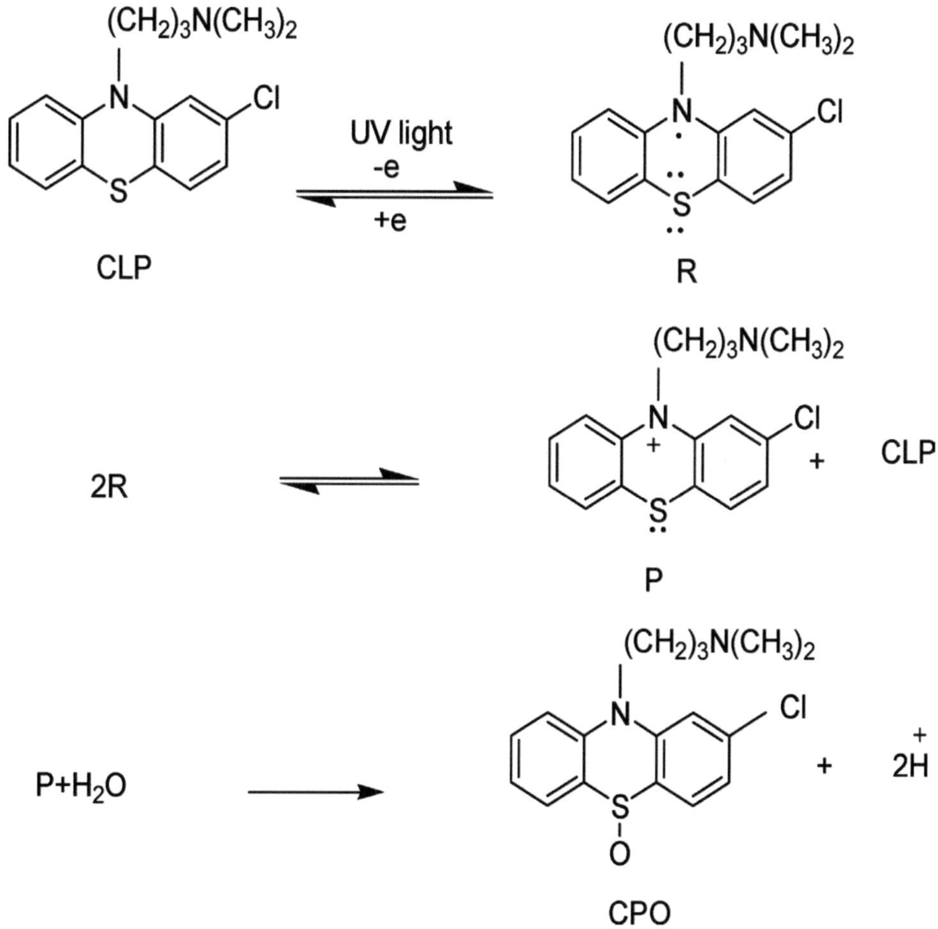

Figure 3.
The effect of ultraviolet light on chlorpromazine (CLP).

The photodegradation of ketoprofen can involve decarboxylation to form an intermediate which then undergoes reduction, or dimerization of the ketoprofen itself.

4. Analytical methods

4.1 Method development

Prior the development of any method for the analysis of certain compound or formulation, there are many factors must be considered before developing the method and applying it to the intended use. The first step include collecting information about the analyte itself (the analyte structure and its physicochemical properties). The mode of detection should be selected (e.g. UV detection). Sample preparation which may include centrifugation, sonication and filtration. The type of the diluent also plays an integral role in the analysis as it should be transparent and does not interfere in the analysis. The stability of the prepared solution, the mobile phase; stationary phase and mode of elution in case of chromatographic elution. All these factors and much more should be considered, optimized and the developed method is then validated and applied for the analysis.

4.2 Spectrophotometric methods

4.2.1 UV/VIS spectrophotometry

Absorption spectrophotometry is the measurement of an interaction between electromagnetic radiation and the molecules, or atoms, of a chemical substance [15]. Techniques frequently employed in pharmaceutical analysis include UV, visible, IR and atomic absorption. Spectrophotometric measurement in the visible region was referred to as colorimetry.

The procedure of UV-unmistakable spectrophotometry includes the estimation of the measure of bright (190–380 nm) or noticeable (380–800 nm) radiation consumed by a substance in arrangement. Retention of light in both the UV and unmistakable area of the electromagnetic range happens when the vitality of the light matches the vitality required to instigate an electronic change and it is related with vibration and rotational progress in the atom. There are two systems of utilizing spectroscopic estimations in medication examination, the total and the similar strategies for measure, and the one utilized relies upon which side of the Atlantic Ocean you complete the investigation. In the UK and Europe the Beer-Lambert condition will in general be utilized in what is known as the outright technique for examine. In this strategy the absorbance is estimated tentatively and the Beer-Lambert condition is comprehended for c, the medication fixation. Hence, the British Pharmacopeia and European Pharmacopeia quote A1% 1 cm qualities in medication monographs. In the US Pharmacopeia, the near strategy for test is liked. In this sort of examine a standard arrangement of the medication to be investigated is readied, the absorbance of the example and the standard are estimated under indistinguishable conditions, and the centralization of the example is determined from the relationship:

$$\frac{\text{Atest}}{[\text{test}]} = \frac{\text{Astd}}{[\text{std}]} \tag{1}$$

Where [test] is the centralization of the example and [std] is the convergence of the readied standard. The relative strategy for test has the bit of leeway that it very well may be utilized regardless of whether the medication experiences a substance response during the measure (for example development of a shaded subsidiary to permit estimation in the obvious district of the range), yet experiences the hindrance that a credible example of the medication being referred to must be accessible for examination. When doing medication examines by spectroscopy it is frequently important to set up a scope of groupings of a standard example of the analyte and measure the absorbance of every arrangement. At the point when these information are plotted, a straight line of positive incline ought to be acquired that goes through the inception. Developing diagrams of this sort not just confirms that the Beer-Lambert law applies to the test at the wavelength of estimation yet additionally enables the chart to be utilized for alignment purposes. An answer of obscure fixation is set up in the very same manner as the benchmarks and its absorbance is estimated at a similar wavelength as the principles. This absorbance is then perused off the alignment chart and the fixation is determined. Standard arrangements arranged independently from the example along these lines are known as outer models. An increasingly thorough system includes the utilization of inside models. An inside standard is an exacerbate that is comparative in compound structure and physical properties to the example being investigated. The inner standard ought to be added to the example being referred to before extraction or measure initiates and is then present in the example framework all through the consequent test. In the measure of complex examples, some example pre-treatment is normally required and the recuperation of the example from the extraction procedure may not be 100%. On the off chance that an inner standard is utilized, misfortunes in test will be reflected by comparative misfortunes in the standard and the proportion of test to standard ought to stay consistent. Inner measures are especially utilized in chromatographic examination (particularly gas chromatography and elite fluid chromatography), where fluctuations in instrumental parameters (for example flow rate of versatile stage) influence precision. In certain spectroscopic examinations a comparable way to deal with the utilization of inner benchmarks is utilized. This is the strategy of standard augmentations and includes expansion of expanding volumes of a standard arrangement of the analyte to a fixed volume of the example and development of an alignment diagram. The diagram in a standard expansion examine is of positive incline however converges they-pivot at a positive estimation of absorbance. The measure of medication in the example is found by extrapolation of the alignment chart back to the point where the line crosses the x-pivot (for example at the point when y 0 in the condition of the line). The strategy for standard increments is generally utilized in nuclear spectroscopy (for example assurance of Ca^{2+} particles in serum by nuclear emanation spectrophotometry) and, since a few aliquots of test are examined to create the alignment chart, should expand the exactness and accuracy of the measure. The chief advantage of colorimetric and spectrophotometric methods is that they provide a simple means for determining minute quantities of substances [16, 17]. Although spectral interference (degradation products, excipients, etc.) can often occur, the selectivity and sensitivity of these methods can be improved by employing an instrumental technique such as derivative spectrophotometry.

4.2.2 Derivative spectrophotometry

In derivative spectrophotometry the absorbance (A) of a sample is differentiated with respect to wavelength (λ) to generate the first, second or higher order derivative [18].

In the context of derivative spectrophotometry, the normal absorption spectrum is referred to as the fundamental, zero order or ^{0}D spectrum.

$A = f(\lambda)$	$dA/d\lambda = f(\lambda)$	$d^2A/\lambda^2 = f\,\Delta(\lambda)$, etc.
Zero order	first order	second derivative

The first derivative (^{1}D) spectrum is a plot of the rate of change of absorbance with wavelength against wavelength, i.e. a plot of the slope of the fundamental spectrum against wavelength. The second derivative (^{2}D) spectrum is a plot of the curvature of the ^{0}D spectrum against wavelength.

The first order derivative spectrum of an absorption band is characterized by a maximum, a minimum and a crossover point at λ_{max} of the absorption band. This bipolar function is characteristic of all odd-order derivatives.

The second derivative spectrum is characterized by two satellite maxima and an inverted band of which the minimum corresponds to the λ_{max} of the fundamental band.

A derivative spectrum is therefore gives better resolution of overlapping bands than the corresponding fundamental spectrum and may permit the accurate determination of the λ_{max} of the individual bands. Secondly, it discriminates in favor of substances of narrow spectral band width against those with broad bandwidth. And consequently, substances with narrow spectral bandwidth display larger derivative amplitude than those with broad bandwidth [15].

These advantages of enhanced resolution and band width discrimination found in derivative spectrophotometry permit the selective determination of certain absorbing substances in samples in which non-specific interference may limit the application of simple spectrophotometric methods. Ephedrine hydrochloride in ephedrine hydrochloride elixir is assayed by second derivative spectrophotometry, which eliminates the broad band absorption of the excipient.

Derivative spectrophotometry has found significant application in clinical, forensic and biomedical analysis. It has been widely applied in the analysis of different pharmaceutical dosage forms. It solves the problem of analysis associated with drug combination, stability studies of drug and degradation products, drug impurities and interference of excipient in drugs [19, 20]. It also solves the problem of analysis of drugs in biological fluids.

4.2.3 Difference spectrophotometry

Both selectivity and accuracy of spectrophotometric analysis of samples, which contain absorbing interferons, may be greatly improved by the technique of difference spectrophotometry. In difference spectrophotometry assays the measured value is the difference in absorbance (ΔA) between two equimolar solutions of the analyte, in different chemical forms which exhibit different spectral characteristics. It is sometimes referred to as differential spectrophotometry.

Certain criteria are required for applying difference spectrophotometry for the analysis of a substance in the presence of other absorbing substances:

1. Reproducible changes are induced in the spectrum of the analyte by the addition of one or more reagents.

2. The absorbance of the interfering substances is not altered by the addition of such reagents.

The simplest and most commonly used techniques for altering the spectral properties of the analyte is the adjustment of the pH of the solution by means of aqueous solution of acids, alkali or buffers [21]. The measured value (ΔA) in a quantitative difference spectrophotometric assay can be proportional to the concentration of the analyte and so it obeys Beer's law. A modified equation may be derived.

$$\Delta A = \Delta abc \qquad (2)$$

Where Δa is the difference absorptivity of the substance at the wavelength of measurement.

The accuracy and selectivity of the method was found to be increased by conversion of normal zero-order or differential UV spectra into higher order [21, 22]. Therefore, the application of difference spectrophotometry is expected to have the totality of advantages of both derivative spectrophotometry (first, second, etc.) combined with delta spectrophotometry [23].

On the other hand, the stability-indicating property, coupled with the selectivity and simplicity of application, of the derivative spectrophotometry (first, second, etc.) and ΔD_1 make these methods more preferable to use for drug analysis than the costly HPLC methods, especially in developing countries.

4.2.4 Colorimetric method

Colorimetric methods, although are generally dependent on functional group in the drug molecule (NH_2, OH, SH), are sometimes utilized as stability-indicating methods. This can be achieved by selectively transforming a drug, its degradation product or its impurity into a derivative so that the spectrum of the derivative is shifted to the visible region.

There are several parameters, which require careful and critical consideration in colorimetry. Firstly, the color reagent should be selective for the drug molecule itself, discriminating degradation products which might be present. Secondly, the effect of any parameters which can affect the development and stability of the color should be established. Moreover, the time required to establish the chromophore should be carefully monitored and assessed.

4.3 Chromatographic methods (HPLC and TLC)

Chromatography is essentially a group of techniques for the separation of the compounds of mixtures by their continuous distribution between two phases. One of the two phases is the fixed (stationary) phase, which can be solid or a liquid supported on a solid. The other phase is a moving (mobile) phase which can be gas or a liquid that flows continuously around the stationary phase.

According to the nature of the mobile phase, chromatography is subdivided into liquid chromatography (LC) where the mobile phase is a liquid, and gas chromatography (GC) where the mobile phase is a gas [15].

4.3.1 Liquid chromatography

There are four classifications for liquid chromatography:

a. Adsorption chromatography: liquid solid chromatography (LSC).

b. Partition chromatography: liquid-liquid chromatography (LLC).

c. Ion exchange chromatography: an ionic liquid mobile phase and a solid polymeric stationary phase containing replaceable ions.

d. Size-exclusion chromatography.

The adsorption and partition chromatography (most widely used in pharmaceutical analysis) are subdivided to:

a. Column chromatography and thin-layer chromatography (TLC): solid stationary phase and liquid mobile phase.

b. Column, paper and thin-layer chromatography: liquid stationary phase and liquid mobile phase.

High performance liquid chromatography (HPLC) belongs to the category of column chromatography and it covers four classes of chromatography: adsorption (LSC), partition (LLC), ion exchange and size-exclusion.

4.3.2 Thin-layer chromatography (TLC)

Thin-layer chromatography has developed into a very sophisticated technique for identification of compounds and for determination of the presence of trace impurities. Separation in TLC occurs by either adsorption or partition. For adsorption, the stationary phase consists of a thin layer of sorbent (e.g. silica) which is activated by heating at 105°C to evaporate water and the mobile phase is devoid of water (usually a mixture of organic solvents).

The term retention time used in TLC is referred to as R_f value which is the distance traveled by the compound from the origin (where the compound is spotted on the plate) divided by the distance traveled by the solvent. Although TLC is widely used for qualitative analysis, it does not in general provide quantitative information of high precision and accuracy. Changes in the practice of TLC have resulted in improved performance of separation and quantitative measurement. These developments are referred to as high-performance thin-layer chromatography (HPTLC) [24].

TLC is widely used in pharmaceutical analysis for:

a. Identification of the components of a mixture by comparing their Rf values with those of reference standard.

b. Detection of any impurities (synthetic route, stability during manufacturing process or storage).

c. Separation of a mixture of compounds and recovery by elution technique.

d. Following synthetic reactions for their completion.

e. Forensic application in drug poisoning or addiction.

4.3.3 High performance liquid chromatography (HPLC)

HPLC is the most commonly used technique for the quantification of drugs in formulations. The principal advantages of HPLC compared to column chromatography are improved resolution of the separated substances, faster separation time and the increased accuracy, precision and sensitivity.

HPLC is based on the same separation modes of column chromatography i.e. adsorption and partition. Unmodified silica (silanol group) is the most widely used in adsorption HPLC. Partition HPLC is divided into two categories, normal-phase and reverse-phase, based on the relative polarities of the stationary and mobile phases.

In order to develop HPLC method and to select the appropriate column type, the analyst needs to know:

a. Suitable solvent for the drug.

b. Molecular structure.

c. Nature of analysis: whether for quantification analysis or stability-indicating method.

The following diagram (**Figure 4**) gives a general guide to the selection of a chromatographic method for separation of compounds of molecular weight $<$ 2000; for samples of higher molecular weight the method of choice would be size-exclusion [25, 26].

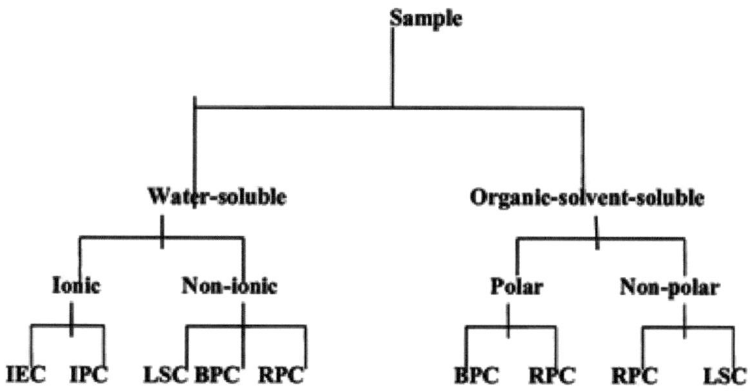

Figure 4.
General guide for selection of chromatographic method.

5. Quality assurance and quality control

In the pharmaceutical Industry, quality management is defined as the aspect of management function that determines and implements the quality policy.

The major elements of quality management are:

a. A quality system describing the organizational structure, procedures, processes and resources.

b. A systematic action or actions necessary to ensure adequate confidence that a product (or service) will satisfy given requirement for quality.

The concepts of quality assurance, GMP and quality control are interrelated aspects of quality management. They are inter-related and have fundamental importance to the production and control of pharmaceutical products.

In fact quality assurance covers quality control in exactly the same manner as it covers other functions such as manufacturing and ware-housing. It approves methods and standards and sees to it that good laboratory practices are operative.

Each manufacturing unit must have a quality control department independent from the production and other departments and under the control of a qualified and experienced personnel and has one or several quality control laboratories at his or her disposal.

Quality control is integral part to all modern industrial processes and the pharmaceutical industry is not an exception. Testing a pharmaceutical product involves physical, chemical and sometimes microbiological analysis. It is a critical function of any business offering a product or service to consumers. In the field of pharmaceutical chemistry, quality control is vital to the successful development, manufacturing, and use of drugs meant to save lives. It determines the quality and stability of drug products via pharmaceutical analysis; it includes areas such as method validation, handling raw materials and finished products, documentations, inspections that impact the development of pharmaceutical products that are governed by specified rules.

Pharmaceutical products are developed and produced according to GMP requirements and other associated codes e.g. good laboratory practices (GLP), and good clinical laboratory practices (GcLP), ... etc.

Production and control operations are clearly specified in a written form i.e. standard operating procedures (SOP's) and GMP requirements are adopted.

Control procedures on starting materials, intermediate products and finished products and other in process controls should be carried out according to written and validated procedures.

The finished products should be correctly processed, checked, packed according to defined procedures.

Finished pharmaceutical products should not be sold or supplied unless they are released by an authorized person.

6. Method validation and statistical interpretation of the analytical method

The function of the analyst is to obtain a result as near to the true value as possible by the correct application of the analytical procedure employed. Quantitative analysis is not simply a case of taking sample, carrying out a single determination and then claim that the value obtained is irrefutable. It also requires knowledge of the chemistry involvements and the possibilities of the interferences from other ions, elements and compounds as well as of the statistical distribution of values [27].

Different errors may occur during the analysis process which should be well noticed and overcome. There are three types of errors:

a. Gross errors: easily recognized as it leads to definite unreliable results: could be due to contaminated reagents, defective instruments, accidental loss of crucial sample etc. It is defined as a serious error so that there is no way to correct the experiment.

b. Random error (in determinate error): the average of the results are very close to the true value, so there is no evidence of bias i.e. some results could be high and some results could be low. Arises from sources that cannot be corrected i.e. the degree of sensitivity of the balance: fourth decimal, fifth decimal. Types of burettes or pipettes (A, B, C types) etc.

c. Systematic (determinant errors): this causes all the results to be in error in the same sense (constant error). May be due to (1) faults in analytical procedure or (2) the equipment used. Observed result could be too low or too high i.e. inaccuracy should be constant (all answers are 10% too high or too low). Example: True value for three samples were 25, 20 and 30% assay result was 35, 30 and 40% respectively i.e. 10% too high. It makes the assay precise but inaccurate sometimes the inaccuracy may be proportional to the true answer, giving rise to proportional error such as 10% of the answer i.e. for the above example for 25% result is 27.5%, 22% for 20% and 33% for30%.

Validation of methods for the quantitative analysis of drugs involves determining as a minimum, their selectivity, and limit of detection, limit of quantification, linearity, working range, accuracy and precision [28].

6.1 Accuracy

Accuracy is a measure of how closely the result of an experiment agrees with the expected result. The difference between the obtained result and the expected result is usually divided by the expected result and reported as a percent relative error [29].

6.2 Precision

Precision is a measure of how close a set of results are to each other [30]. It is often measured under repeatable (same analyst, same day, same instruments and same materials) and reproducible conditions. Precision always accompanies accuracy, but a high degree of precision does not imply accuracy.

6.3 Linearity

For any developed analytical method, standard curve is constructed to verify the linear relationship between the concentration and a characteristic parameter for a component such as peak area, peak height or peak ratio in chromatographic analysis or UV-absorption in spectrophotometry.

Most analytical methods are based on processes where the method produces a response that is linear and which increases or decreases linearly with analyte concentration. In other words, it is the ability of the method to elicit test results that directly proportional to the concentration of analyte within a given range.

Statistical application is important in evaluating calibration graphs in instrumental analysis. The equation of a straight line takes the form:

$$y = a + bx \qquad (3)$$

Where a is the intercept of the straight line with the y axis and b is the slope of the line.

The statistical measure of the goodness of the fit of the line through the data is the correlation coefficient "r". It falls in the range $-1 \leq r \geq +1$. Negative r-values indicate negative slope and vice-versa. It is important to note that calculated r-values can be sometimes misleading and a calibration curve must be physically plotted to ensure the shape of the plot. From the calculated regression line data, the concentration of the analyte can be estimated by interpolation. Each value of y is subjected to random error and likely an error in the slope and intercept values can occur. This can be resolved by calculating standard deviations of the slope (S_b) and intercept (S_a). S_b and S_a are obtained from a calculated statistic value $S_{y/x}$ [29]. The values of S_b and S_a are used to calculate the confidence limits for the slope and intercept using a *t*-value at a desired confidence level, normally 95% level. These limits are important to indicate if there is a significant difference between these values and certain true values, which reflects the effect of random or systemic errors.

6.4 Limit of detection

The limit of detection is the lowest content of analyte that can be distinguished from background noise and measured with reasonable statistical certainty. It can be calculated by the reduced formula:

$$3SB/b \qquad (4)$$

Where SB = Sy/x (calculated from the regression analysis data), b is slope [29].

6.5 Limit of quantification

The lower limit of quantification is the amount equal to or greater than the lowest concentration point on the calibration curve that can be measured with an acceptable level of accuracy and precision [29].

It can be calculated by the equation:

$$10SB/b \qquad (5)$$

Where SB = Sy/x (calculated from the regression analysis data), b is slope.

6.6 Method comparison

The comparison of two methods should be carried out using a suitable statistical procedure to test if there are significant differences between them. The *t*-test provides a simple check on accuracy and the *F*-test on precision. These tests require the knowledge of what is known as the number of degrees of freedom.

7. Conclusion

Pharmaceutical products must be analyzed regularly to ensure their safety and effectiveness. This chapter described the quality assurance and quality control of materials and finished products. The requirements to develop a suitable method and its validation. Also different analytical methods and their application in the field of pharmaceutical analysis was also discussed.

Conflict of interest

The author declares that there is no conflict of interest.

Author details

Shaza W. Shantier
Department of Pharmaceutical Chemistry, Faculty of Pharmacy, University of Khartoum, Sudan

*Address all correspondence to: sshantier@yahoo.com

References

[1] Blass B. Basic Principles of Drug Discovery and Development. 1st ed. Amsterdam: Academic Press; 2015

[2] Cairns D. Essentials of Pharmaceutical Chemistry. 3rd ed. UK: Pharmaceutical Press; 2008

[3] Jeffery GH, Bassett J, Mendham J, Denney RC. Vogel's Textbook of Quantitative Chemical Analysis. 5th ed. England, UK: Longman Scientific and Technical; 1989

[4] Aulton ME. The Science of Dosage Forms Design. 2nd ed. Toronto: Churchill Livingstoe; 2002. p. 129

[5] Florence AT, Attwood D. Physicochemical Properties of Pharmacy, Chapter 4. 4th ed. Chicago, London: Pharmaceutical Press; 2006

[6] Genaro AR. Remington, The Science and Practice of Pharmacy. 20th ed. Philadelphia: Lippincott Williams and Wilkins; 2000. p. 986

[7] Ansel HC, Popovich NG, Allen LV. Pharmaceuticals Dosage Forms and Drug Delivery Systems. 6th ed. Philadelphia: Williams and Wilkins; 1995. p. 117

[8] Lund W. The Pharmaceutical Codex. Principles and Practice of Pharmaceutics. 12th ed. London: Pharmaceutical Press; 1994. pp. 69, 277, 283

[9] Carstensen JT. Drug Stability Principles and Practices. 2nd ed. New York: Marcel Deckker; 1995. p. 91

[10] Grossweiner LI. Photophysics. In: Smith KC, editor. The Science of Photobiology. New York: Plenum Press; 1989. p. 12

[11] Cadet J, Anselmino C, Douki T, Voituriez L. Photochemistry of nucleic acid in cells. Journal of Photochemistry and Photobiology B: Biology. 1992;**15**:277

[12] Albini A, Fasani E. Drugs Photochemistry and Photostability. Cambridge: The Royal Society of Chemistry; 1998. pp. 29, 54, 132, 171

[13] Greenhill JV, McLelland MA. Photodecomposition of drugs. Progress in Medicinal Chemistry. 1990;**27**:51-121

[14] Tonnesen HH. Photostability of Drugs and Drug Formulations. London: Tylor and Francis; 1996. pp. 5-121

[15] Beckett AH, Stenlake JB. Practical Pharmaceutical Chemistry. 4th ed. UK: Athlone Press; 2004. pp. 260, 296-300

[16] Shantier SW, Gadkariem EA, Ibrahim KAE. A colorimetric method for the determination of tobramycin. International Journal of Drug Formulation and Research. 2011;**2**(4):260-272

[17] Shantier SW, Gadkriem EA. Colorimetric methods for determination of cefquinome sulphate. American Journal of Applied Sciences. 2014;**11**(2):202-206

[18] Anthony CM, Widdop B, Moss MS. Clarck's Isolation and Identification of Drugs. 2nd ed. UK: The Pharmaceutical Press; 2006

[19] Shantier SW, Gadkriem EA, Adam MO, Mohamed MA. Development of stability-indicating methods for cefquinome sulphate. International Journal of Biomedical Sciences. 2013;**9**(3):161-167

[20] Elimam MM, Shantier SW, GadkariemEA,MohamedMA.Derivative spectrophotometric methods for the analysis and stability studies of

colistin sulphate. Journal of Chemistry. 2015;**2015**:5. Article ID 624316

[21] Davidson AG, Hassan SV. Assay of benzenoid drugs in tablet and capsule formulations by second-derivative ultraviolet spectrophotometry. Journal of Pharmaceutical Sciences. 1984;**73**:413

[22] Abounassif MA. pH-Induced difference spectrophotometric assay of bromazepam. Journal de Pharmacie de Belgique. 1989;**44**:329

[23] ShantierSW,GadkriemEA.Differential spectrophotometric method for determination of cefquinome sulphate. British Journal of Pharmaceutical Research. 2014;**4**(5):617-625

[24] Yuri K, Rosario L. HPLC for Pharmaceutical Scientists. Hoboken, New Jersey: John Wiley and Sons; 2007

[25] Veronika RM. Practical High-Performance Liquid Chromatography. 3rd ed. New York: John Wiley and Sons; 1999. p. 15

[26] Watson DG. Pharmaceutical Analysis. 2nd ed. UK: Harcourt Publishers Limited; 1999. pp. 80, 90-92, 238, 278

[27] Harvey D. Modern Analytical Chemistry. USA: The McGraw-Hill Companies; 2000. p. 38

[28] ICH Harmonized Tripartite Guideline, Stability Testing of New Drug Substances and Products; 2003. pp. 1-15

[29] Miller JC, Miller JN. Statistics and Chemometrics for Analytical Chemistry. 5th ed. England: Pearson Education; 2005

[30] Robinson JW. Undergraduate Instrumental Analysis. 5th ed. New York, Basel: Marcel Dekker; 1995. p. 16

Chapter 3

Microcrystalline Cellulose as Pharmaceutical Excipient

Anis Yohana Chaerunisaa, Sriwidodo Sriwidodo and Marline Abdassah

Abstract

Microcrystalline cellulose (MCC) is a pure partially depolymerized cellulose synthesized from α-cellulose precursor (type Iβ), obtained as a pulp from fibrous plant material, with mineral acids using hydrochloric acid to reduce the degree of polymerization. The MCC can be synthesized by different processes such as reactive extrusion, enzyme mediated, steam explosion, and acid hydrolysis. It is commonly manufactured by spray-drying the neutralized aqueous slurry of hydrolyzed cellulose. The MCC is a valuable additive in pharmaceutical, food, cosmetic, and other industries. MMC obtained from different sources will differ considerably in chemical composition, structural organization, and physicochemical properties (crystallinity, moisture content, surface area and porous structure, molecular weight, etc.). The high demand of microcrystalline cellulose used in pharmaceutical industries has led to the utilization of locally and naturally occurring materials in the production of microcrystalline cellulose. Many studies on the physicochemical properties of locally produced MCC derived from natural sources have been extensively evaluated in the development of a new natural source for MCC as a substitution of wood, the most abundant one.

Keywords: microcrystalline cellulose, excipient, MCC, filler, Avicel

1. Introduction

Cellulose, a fibrous carbohydrate found in all plants, is the most abundant natural polymer with biomass production of 50 billion tons per year [1]. Cellulose is a linear polymer of glucose. Based on solubility in alkaline, cellulose is divided into three groups which are alpha, beta, and gamma celluloses. Microcrystalline cellulose (MCC) is a purified, partially depolymerized cellulose having the formula $(C_6H_{10}O_5)_n$. It is prepared by treating alpha cellulose with mineral acids (type Ib). This polysaccharide polymer consists of a linear chain of several hundred to over ten thousand β(1 → 4) linked D-glucose units, consisting of linear chains of *β*-1,4-D anhydroglucopyranosyl units. Raw material used for MMC preparation is a pulp from a fibrous plant such as conifer wood. Cotton is also a possible cellulose source for MCC [2, 3]. Pharmaceutical grade MCC, which needs a high-quality pulp, used wood as the most common source. From such wooden source, cellulose chains are packed in layers and held together by strong hydrogen bonds from lignin, a cross-linking polymer. For that purpose, both softwoods (evergreen conifer) and hardwoods (deciduous broadleaf) can be used [4]. These woods differ not only in chemical composition including cellulose proportions, hemicelluloses, and lignin but also in structural organization, i.e., regions which are relatively more crystalline or amorphous. The amorphous regions are more prone to hydrolysis by acid resulting in shorter and more crystalline fragments.

Non-woody lignocellulosic materials have also been developed as source of MCC such as cotton linters [5], cotton stalks [6], cotton rags [5], cotton fabric waste [7], cotton wool [8], soybean husk [9], corn cob [10], water hyacinth [11], coconut shells [12], oil palm biomass residue [13, 14], oil palm fronds [15], rice husk [6, 16], sugar cane bagasse [6, 16–20], jute [21, 22], ramie [23], fibers and straw of flax [24], wheat straw [25], sorghum stalks [26], sisal fibers [27] and mangosteen [28], alfa grass fibers [29, 30], soybean hulls [31], orange mesocarp [32], Indian bamboo [33], roselle fiber [34], and alfa fiber [35]. Seed flosses from milkweed pods (*Calotropis procera*), shrubs, and kapok (*Ceiba pentandra*) trees are also known as cellulosic resources. Due to its high purity of alpha cellulose, most seed flosses must be treated to remove impurities including lignin, pectin, and wax [36].

Wooden sources contain cellulose chains which are packed as layers held by cross-linking hydrogen bonds [37]. Chemically it consists of polymeric matrix of lignin, hemicelluloses, and pectin [38]. Different woods considerably possessed different chemical composition of cellulose (including allocations of cellulose, hemicelluloses, and lignin in cell wall) and structural organization as well. Relatively different crystallinity in particular regions is observed as more amorphous according to softwoods (evergreen conifer) and hardwoods which are termed as deciduous broadleaf [4, 37]. The amorphous regions of cellulose provide a more susceptible property for depolymerization by acid hydrolysis. At optimum acid concentration, the process gave shorter and more crystalline fragments such as the MCC [2, 37].

2. Synthesis of MCC

The MCC can be synthesized by different processes including extrusion and enzyme-mediated process [25]. Other studies reported that it can also be synthesized by steam explosion and acid hydrolysis process [5, 6]. The acid hydrolysis process is more preferable due to shorter duration than others. It also offered the possibility to be applied as a continuous process rather than a batch-type process. Limited quantity of consumed acid is also the advantage of the process, while, despite the lower unit cost from less chemicals used, this process offered more fine particles of the MCC as the final product [5]. Fibrous plant pulp is hydrolyzed by mineral acid under heat and pressure. In the presence of water and acid, hydrolysis process breaks cellulose polymers into smaller chain polymers or microcrystals. Other celluloses, to which soluble components of cellulose such as beta and gamma celluloses, hemicelluloses, and lignin are dissolved with acid and water, are separated out during washing process by water which continued by filtration. The obtained pure alpha cellulose has then been neutralized and given the slurry final product [3]. This suspension is dried to obtain the insoluble white, odorless, tasteless powder, which has later been characterized as MCC [39]. MCC is hygroscopic in nature, and insoluble in water, but swells when in contact with water.

Another synthesis procedure of the MCC reported by Ohwoavworhua et al. [40] can be concluded as follows: the α-cellulose was hydrolyzed with hydrochloric acid at a boiling temperature of 105° for 15 min. The neutralized slurry obtained from the hydrolysis process was washed, and the fraction passing through 710 μm sieve was stored at room temperature in a desiccator. MCC is commonly dried from the slurry by spray-drying method. By varying spray-drying conditions, the degree of agglomeration and moisture content can be manipulated. In order to obtain smaller particle sizes (below 50 μm), further milling MCC can be performed [1].

Other drying techniques may be used, which may require additional screening steps postdrying in order to control particle size distribution [41, 42]. Higher bulk density grades are also available by using specific cellulose pulps (raw material), and median particle sizes below 50 mm can be obtained by further milling MCC [1].

Several studies have compared microcrystalline cellulose with various sources, including different manufacturers and different sites [4, 43–47]. MCC produced by various manufacturers or in various manufacturing sites may have different properties due to the kinds of pulp used as raw materials and their respective manufacturing conditions [2, 4]. A number of studies have confirmed that the moisture content of MCC influences compaction properties, tensile strength, and viscoelastic properties [48].

Type	Conc.	Hydrolysis condition		MCC-Y (%)	Duration (minute)	References
		L/C (vol./wt)	Temperature (°C)			
HCl	2 N	10:1	105	15	n.a	[5]
HCl	2 N	10:1	45	15	n.a	[6]
HCl	2.5 N	20:1	85	90	80	[5]
HCl	2.5 N	62.5:1	105	15	19	[6]
HCl	2 N	10:1	n.a	45–60	n.a	[7]

Table 1.
Hydrolysis reagents (acid type and concentration), liquor to cellulose ratio (L/C), hydrolysis conditions, and yield of microcrystalline cellulose (MCC-Y) hydrolysis reagent.

MCC Type	Particle size (micron)	Utilization
PH 101	50	It is most widely used for direct compression tableting, for wet granulation, for spheronization, and in capsule filling processes
PH 102	100	It is used as the PH-101, but its larger particle size improves the flow of fine powders
PH 103	50	It has the same particle size as PH-101 with lower moisture content (3%), so it is used for moisture-sensitive pharmaceutical active ingredients
PH 105	Less than 50	It is the most compressible of the PH products owing the smallest particle size. Well known as excipient for direct compression for granular or crystalline materials. When mixed with PH-101 or PH-102, specific flow and compression characteristics will be obtained. It has applications in roller compaction
PH 112	100	It has the same particle size as PH-102. It has lower moisture content (1.5%). It is used for high moisture-sensitive pharmaceutical active ingredients
PH 113	50	It has the same particle size as PH-101. It has lower moisture content (1.5%). It is used for high moisture-sensitive pharmaceutical active ingredients
PH 200	180	It has a large particle size with increased flowability. It is used to reduce weight variation and to improve content uniformity in direct compression formulations and in wet granulation formulations
PH 301	50	It has the same particle size as PH-101 but is denser providing more flowability and tablet weight uniformity. Useful for making smaller tablets and in capsule filling excipient

Table 2.
Types of the commercial microcrystalline cellulose [1, 51].

It was generally recognized that batch-to-batch variability from a sole manufacturing site was less important than differences observed between multiple sources. Only a few studies have tried to correlate the manufacturing conditions of microcrystalline cellulose with its physicochemical properties and its performance in tableting applications [2, 49, 50]. The effect of some parameters on hydrolysis process on yield value of production is shown in **Tables 1** and **2**.

3. Physicochemical properties of MCC

3.1 Moisture content

A number of studies have confirmed that the moisture content of MCC influences compaction properties, tensile strength, and *viscoelastic* properties [48, 52, 53]. Moisture within the pores of MCC may act as an internal lubricant, reduce frictional forces, and facilitate slippage and plastic flow within the individual microcrystals [54, 55]. The lubricating properties of water may also reduce tablet density variation by providing a better transmission of the compression force through the compact and by decreasing the adhesion of the tablet to the die wall [55, 56]. Compressibility of MCC depends on moisture content, which means that when MCC having different moisture content is compressed with the same pressure, it may not result in the same compact porosity. It is very well known that compaction pressure required to produce certain porosity (or solid fraction) decreases with increasing moisture content. Sun reported that below 3% water content, the compaction properties of MCC were insensitive to variation of moisture [53]. However up to an optimum level, an increase of moisture will increase the tablet strength of most excipients. This can be explained by the fact that molecular binding in water vapor layers reduces interparticular surface distances, hence increasing intermolecular attraction forces [56].

The storage conditions of the MCC compacts also play an important role, as an increase in relative humidity will negatively impact tablet strength [47]. However this softening is often reversible when tablets are removed from the humid environment [1]. Fundamental forces affecting powder flow are cohesion and friction [55]. Frictional forces and electrostatic charges between particles during the compression process will decrease as moisture content increases. Moisture may also play a role in increasing cohesion forces inside particles due to the creation of liquid or even solid bridges. In the case of MCC as excipient, significant changes in flowability were observed when increasing moisture contents were applied which resulted in changes in powder cohesiveness. This phenomenon was described by the increase in compressibility index and the shear cell [48].

3.2 Particle size

Particle size has a very little effect on the tabletability of neat MCC, i.e., not lubricated nor blended with other excipients or active pharmaceutical ingredients (APIs) [57–60]. MCC particle size and moisture content are often considered as the most important CMAs for tableting performance [61]. Considering that the brittle-ductile transition diameter (Dcrit) of MCC is 1949 mm, standard MCC grades, having particle sizes below Dcrit, should all deform plastically when compression pressure exceeds yield pressure. Coarser grades of MCC, characterized by a smaller envelope surface area, have been reported to be more lubricant sensitive than finer MCC [52, 58, 62, 63]. In complete formulations finer MCCs would therefore promote tablet (compact) strength [64, 65]. Reducing the particle size of MCC will increase cohesiveness and hence as a consequence surely affect its flowability. Kushner et al. reported that different particle sizes of excipient may impact tablet characteristics including hardness, friability, disintegration, and content uniformity [66]. Improved flowability will be obtained when coarser MCCs are employed as well as reduction in tablet weight variation [67]. Hlinak et al. suggested that particle size may also impact wetting properties, dissolution of the API, and stability of drug products [68].

Albers et al. evaluated the tableting properties of three batches from five different brands MCC type 101 [43]. Batches using single manufacturer source produced more similar tablet characteristic than those using samples from various sources. Statistically significant differences were also observed within single brands of MCC. From a different batch of MCC studied, the greatest differences in powder properties were observed in the median particle size and specific surface area. Despite the lower median particle size of Avicel PH-101 (FMC), this MCC was described as easy flowing powder compared to other brands as illustrated by its low compressibility index and high values of shear cell flow functions (FFc) which exceed 4.

Williams et al. used tableting indices to investigate the compaction properties of MCC types 101 and 102 (median particle size of about 50 and 100 mm, respectively), each type being represented by two batches from five different sources [47]. The lubricant sensitivity of MCC expressed as its compressibility decreased when this excipient was mixed with other materials such as magnesium stearate. Another factor affecting lubricant sensitivity of MCC is the particle size. A higher particle size of MCC, Avicel PH-200 (180 microns), is more sensitive to lubricant than Avicel PH-101 (50 microns). At the same concentration, the lubricant covers more efficiently a larger particle size of MCC (PH-200) than that of the smaller particle size of MCC (PH-101) due to a larger particle surface area of smaller particles of MCC [51].

Compactability of the MCC particles is affected by the porosity. Avicel PH-101, Avicel PH-102, and Avicel PH-200 as marketed products of MCC owing almost the same density showed the same compressibility despite their mean particle size which varies from 50 to 180 microns. Avicel PH-301 (50 microns) and Avicel PH-302 (90 microns) which physically are more dense revealed less compressible or compactable properties [51].

3.3 Particle morphology

Obae et al. suggested that MCC morphology, described by the length of particles (L) and their width (D), was one of the most important factors influencing tabletability [69]. Rod-shaped particles which are fibrous and having higher L/D ratios resulted in higher tablet strengths than round-shaped particles. Other physicochemical properties of MCC including moisture content, bulk density, and specific surface area did not correlate well with tensile strength of obtained tablet. Obae et al. illustrated the reduction of bulk density and flowability and the increase of specific surface area when the L/D ratio increased. This may be due to the property of the particles which is more fibrous. MCC morphology was found to be affecting the drug dissolution which may due to porosity [70].

3.4 Crystallinity

Modifying the hydrolysis conditions, including temperature, time, and acid concentration, also has a very little impact on the degree of crystallinity, i.e., the regularity of the arrangement of the cellulose polymer chains [2, 50]. This observation indicates that crystallinity cannot be controlled at the hydrolysis stage. Crystallinity appears to be more dependent on pulp source rather than on processing conditions [4], which is consistent with the method of MCC manufacture where the acid preferentially attacks the (pulp dependent) amorphous regions.

The total amount of sorbed water in MCC is proportional to the fraction of amorphous material [48, 54, 55]. Therefore MCC powders with a lower degree of crystallinity may contain more water than their counterparts with a higher degree. If low-crystallinity MCC preferentially binds more water, moisture-sensitive APIs may exhibit lower rates of degradation [71]. Despite the controversial impact of crystallinity, it may influence the adsorption of water on cellulose microfibrils, which may in turn influence flowability, tabletability, and stability of the drug product.

3.5 Bulk density

Mostly, direct compression excipients are spray-dried; therefore porous structure was produced as a result. This property is characterized by a relatively low bulk density. Increase in porosity (lower density) facilitates higher compressibility, i.e., the densification of a powder bed due to the application of a stress [56]. The improved compressibility of plastically deforming materials, such as MCC, might then result in improved tabletability as a result of the increased bonding surface area [72]. The higher roughness of low density MCC particles may also contribute to particle interlocking [73]. Low bulk density MCC will provide higher dilution potential and hence better counteract the poor tableting properties of APIs. Granulation or drying as preprocesses of tablet formulation will densify MCC hence less tabletable than the original porous MCC [74, 75]. It can therefore be generalized that a decrease in bulk density improves tabletability; however, it will often hinder flowability [62].

3.6 Degree of polymerization

The degree of polymerization (DP) expresses the number of glucose units ($C_6H_{10}O_5$) in the cellulose chain. It decreases exponentially as a function of hydrolysis conditions, including temperature, acid concentration, and time of reaction. The rate of hydrolysis slows down to a certain value which is stated as level-off degree of polymerization (LODP). The LODP value is specific for a particular pulp, and it is usually between the range of 200 and 300 [44, 61], e.g., 180–210 range for hardwood pulps and 210–250 for softwood pulps. Theoretically, to obtain a certain degree of polymerization which is higher than the LODP value, hydrolysis process could be terminated at any time. However, due to the exponential decay of DP, this termination is neither a robust nor a reproducible approach. The degree of polymerization is used as an identity test, as pharmacopoeial MCC is defined by a DP below 350 glucose units, compared to DPs in the order of 10,000 units for the original native cellulose [1].

The correlation between the degree of polymerization (DP) of MCC and its tabletability has not been explored yet. Therefore, it is merely an identity test to distinguish the tabletability of MCC (DP < 350) compared with powdered cellulose (DP > 440). Dybowski showed that the origin of the raw materials and the production method of MCC more decisively influence the physical characteristics than DP. DP value is a criterion used to guide the manufacturer about hydrolysis of MCC, whereas for the user it is a characteristic to distinguish between properties of MCC and powdered cellulose.

Wood pulps with high bulk density grades which can be characterized by lower level-off DP should not be directly compared with standard grades. This parameter reflects the lack of distinction between the degree of polymerization (DP) and level-off degree of polymerization (LODP). LODP is typical of a particular raw material, with a common value between the range of 200 and 300 [44]. Cellulose having LODP value at this range usually difficult for further hydrolysis. In contrast, cellulose materials with DP values higher than the level-off degree of polymerization plateau are more difficult to control due to their greater sensitivity to hydrolysis. Owing LODP above 200–300, the MCC remains to be more fibrous, which would result in a lower bulk density, with improved tabletability, but would hinder powder flow [49, 50]. Below the LODP MCC is less fibrous, denser, and less tabletable. Tabletability is not related to a particular DP value; as an example powdered cellulose has a higher DP than MCC but is not as tabletable [1].

3.7 Effect of lignin

Landín et al. compared four brands of MCC [45]. Different woods used as raw materials, i.e., hardwood versus softwood, suggested differences in lignin and hemicelluloses composition. The non-cellulose component has also significantly different manufacturing process intensities which resulted in variable suggestive composition and potentially varying qualities of product. Landín et al. found that lignin content increased the dissolution rate of prednisone [46]. Lignin being hydrophobic may alter cellulose–cellulose and/or cellulose–API interactions and hence drug release rate.

Thoorens et al. [37] studied that differences in packing and flow properties which are shown by scanning electron micrographs from Avicel PH-101 and Avicel PH-102 were attributed to differences in moisture content, particle shape, and particle size distribution. Tabletability which also varied among the MCC samples were attributed to the differences in moisture content and the internal structure of the particles. These are mostly caused by different processing conditions which are specific to each manufacturer. However, the impacts of crystallinity and particle morphology are negligible. Significant differences in lubricant sensitivity, compressibility, and tablet disintegration were also noted between MCCs due to various manufacturing processes by different manufacturers. Variability between lots from the same manufacturer was found to give a smaller effect on properties of MCC product. A current study from Doelker concluded that even if all of various MCCs comply with compendial specifications, large differences still exist among them [44].

4. MCC as pharmaceutical excipients

According to the International Pharmaceutical Excipient Council (IPEC), excipients are the process aids or any substances other than the active pharmaceutical ingredient that are included in pharmaceutical dosage forms. The functionalities of excipient are to impart weight, consistency, and volume which allow accuracy of dose, improve solubility, and in the end increase stability. It can also be proposed to enhance bioavailability, modifying drug release and used in product quick identification, increase patient acceptability, and facilitate dosage form design.

Excipients classified as:

1. Primary excipients: diluents (filler), binders (adhesives), disintegrants, lubricants, antiadhesives, glidants

2. Secondary excipients: coloring agents, flavors, sweeteners, coating agents, plasticizers wetting agents, buffers, and adsorbents

Diluents are incorporated into tablet or capsule dosage forms to increase dosage form volume or weight and can also be referred as fillers. Direct compression binders are functional even at low use levels and offer superior tabletability [1]. Some diluents, such as microcrystalline cellulose, can also be considered as dry binders since they improve the compactibility or tabletability of the compression mix.

Microcrystalline cellulose, according to many publications, is an excipient of outstanding merit and remains the most widely used direct compression excipient serving as a strong dry binder, tablet disintegrant, an absorbent, filler or diluent, a lubricant, and anti-adherent.

MCC is generally considered as the diluent having the best binding properties and is recognized as one of the preferred DC binders [44, 76]. It is used as a binder/diluent in oral tablet and capsule formulations including both wet granulation and direct compression processes. It also has some lubricant and disintegrant properties which is useful in direct tableting. Small amounts of MCCs are able to efficiently bind other materials, especially poorly tabletable active pharmaceutical ingredients. MCC exhibits a high dilution potential, whereas the broad particle size range provides optimum packing density and coverage of other materials [44, 54].

MCC has been the most favorite diluent among others due to its low bulk density. Excipient having low bulk density and large particle size distribution will exhibit a high dilution potential on a weight basis, optimum packing density, and coverage of drug and other excipient materials [77].

MCC is commercially available in different particle sizes, density, and moisture grades that have different properties and applications. The most widely pronounced grades are Avicel PH 101 and Avicel PH 102 (FMC Corporation, Princeton, NJ, USA). PH stands for the pharmaceutical grade of MCC. Avicel PH 101 is the original grade of MCC, while PH 102 is available as a partially agglomerated product with a larger particle size distribution and slightly better fluidity. Both grades show no significant difference in the compressibility [78].

4.1 MCC as directly compressible filler

MCC has been very well known as the most compressible of all direct compression fillers which has the highest dilution potential and capacity. It is defined as the amount of active ingredient that a diluent can successfully carry in the direct compression method. This property can be explained by the basis of the physicochemical nature of MCC particles, which are held together by hydrogen bonds. MCC particles are deformed plastically under compaction forces to yield an extremely large number of clean surfaces brought in contact during this deformation, forming a strong compact even under low compression forces [78].

Direct compression (DC) is the tableting process of a blend of ingredients without a preliminary granulation or agglomeration process. Despite involving only few process steps, product design in DC can be challenging because of the numerous competing objectives [79]. Direct compression requires increased performance, quality, and consistency from the starting ingredients including excipients [44, 56, 80, 81]. The use of poorly controlled or inadequately specified raw materials may lead to several challenges in DC, such as poor flowability and inconsistent tablet weight, unsatisfactory tablet strength, lack of content uniformity or segregation, and dissolution failure [56, 82, 83]. Among several requirements, the compression mix has to flow to ensure a consistent tablet weight; it has to compress and compact into robust tablets. Overall, as a direct compression filler, Avicel promotes efficient dry blending of ingredients and produces tablets with high hardness levels and low friability levels with excellent compression. It produces tablets of superior whiteness and color stability.

Lately, MCC can be considered as the most widely used diluent in the direct compression and wet granulated tablet making procedures. MCC type 102, having a median particle size of about 100 mm (D50 value measured by laser diffraction), presents acceptable flow properties required for successful high-speed tableting [2, 84]. However due to the low bulk density of MCC, its mass flow is less than that of other common and denser excipients such as direct compression grades of lactose or dibasic calcium phosphates [43, 44, 59, 82]. Avicel grades (Avicel PH-102 SCG, Avicel HFE-102, Avicel PH-200, Avicel PH-302) provide excipient solutions to many challenges of direct compression formulations including improved flow, better compressibility, and accommodation of moisture-sensitive actives [78]. The larger particle size grades generally provide better flow properties, while low-moisture grades are used for moisture-sensitive materials. Higher-density grades have improved flowability. Flowability may be improved by selecting coarser grades of MCC with a larger number of aggregates, such as MCC type 200 with a median particle size approximating 200 mm [58, 85].

The difference between these common excipients is less pronounced on a volumetric basis [86], which determines die fill. Another approach may be to combine MCC with other free flowing excipients or glidants [59, 62, 87]. Gamble et al. observed that the particle size distributions of coarser grades of MCC do not scale up proportionally [58]. MCC types 101, 102, and 200 all have primary particles of about 50 mm but differ in the number of larger aggregated particles. These aggregates, accounting for a large volume/mass fraction but a low number fraction, enable improved flow.

During compression, MCC plastically deforms and therefore maximizes the area of interparticle bonding [88]. Mechanical interlocking of irregularly shaped and elongated MCC particles has also been suggested to enhance tabletability [44, 60, 75]. The plasticity of MCC is the main reason of its exceptional binding properties. However, compared to brittle excipients, MCC is more lubricant sensitive. For a constant number of revolutions, tabletability may also decrease with increasing blender sizes and decreasing loadings in the blender [89]. The viscoelastic behavior of MCC also explains its strain rate sensitivity (SRS), which refers to the greater elastic effects at higher tableting speeds where there is insufficient compaction time for plastic deformation [90]. The strain rate sensitivity of viscoelastic excipients has to be taken into account by the formulation scientists in order to design robust formulations.

4.2 MCC as wet granulation filler

MCC is one of the types of filler which is water insoluble having swelling tendencies and excellent water imbibing or wicking action. Other filler examples with the same property are calcium pectinate and sodium alginate. This property makes MCC as also an excipient of choice for wet granulation. Both Avicel PH 101 and Avicel PH 102 can be used advantageously as fillers in wet granulation in a concentration of 5.15%. When used as filler in wet granulation method, the wicking action of MCC promotes rapid wetting of the powder mix. Another advantage offfered by using MCC as wet granulation filler is the ability to retain water, which makes the wet mass less sensitive to overwetting due to an excess of granulating fluid. The milling of the wet mass will be much easier due to less clogging of the screen; hence it will produce a more uniform granules. Drying process also will be more homogeneous, and the case of hardening can be reduced. Case hardening is a phenomenon which is observed in incompletely dried granules. This case happened when the granules are dried at a high temperature, from which the inside part of the granules remains wet, while the surface seems dried. The granules are often hard and resist disintegration. When coming to compaction process, the compression forces will break the granules and deform plastically to form soft tablets due to the moisture coming out of the incompletely dried granules. The use of Avicel PH 101 or Avicel PH 302 as filler in wet granulation promotes rapid wetting as a result of the wicking action of MCC. They reduce sensitivity of the wet mass to overwetting and increase the drying process speed. Since there is fewer excess of granulating fluid, screen blockages and case hardenings can be reduced. Homogeneous and uniform granule when MCC is used as wet granulation filler will reduce dye migration. When MCC is employed, faster disintegration from granules and tablets will be obtained.

4.2.1 Benefits of MCC in wet granulation

Basically, using MCC in wet granulation included wetting MCC with water followed by drying and compression. The process resulted in lower hardness tablets than that with dry compression. The wet granulation reduces the density of agglomerated particles thereby decreasing their internal surface area. In contrast, it can also cause adhesion between particle agglomerates, reducing external surface area resulting in less particle interlocking and hydrogen bonding. In general, using Avicel PH-101 or Avicel PH-102 in wet granulation formulations with concentration between 5 and 20% offers the following benefits [51]:

1. Rapid adsorption of water by MCC and distribution through the mixture

2. Decrease of sensitivity to water content, wet screening, and localized overwetting due to the large surface area of MCC, hence high adsorptive capacity

3. Increased drying efficiency

4. Decreased color mottling

5. Better drug content uniformity

6. Higher tablet hardness at the same compression force with less friability

4.3 Filler in dry granulation

Roller compaction is a dry process involving compaction of materials that are then milled to generate a granulation. This granulation is then lubricated and compressed on a tablet machine. This process can be used for moisture-sensitive active pharmaceutical ingredients. The use of Avicel PH grades in roller compaction includes improvement of compaction in the ribbon phase, enhancement of flow of the granules, and preserving of the content uniformity of the Þ nal granulation.

4.4 MCC as binder

MCC is a self-disintegrating binder [91] with low lubricant requirement with regard to its dry binding properties due to the extreme low coefficient of friction and its very low residual die wall pressure [56, 62, 92]. However these properties do not replace the need for true disintegrants and lubricants as an addition when MCC is used in a tablet formulation. In fact combination of MCC and superdisintegrants may be complementary to promote fast disintegration [93, 94]. Other advantages of MCC include broad compatibility with various APIs, physiological inertness, ease of handling, and ease of supply for manufacturer [54].

Study on the use of MCC with spray-dried lactose as the poorest compressibility among all directly compressible fillers showed that a blend of 200 mg of spray-dried lactose with appropriate lubricants may not be able to compress unless a correct amount of dry binder is incorporated inside the blend. Incorporation of 2.5% of Avicel to the formulation proved that MCC has served the purpose. A number of Avicel such as PH-113 can act as a dry binder [95]. However, it will also function as a disintegrant when dry compression is employed.

4.4.1 MCC as a wet binder

MCC can also be used as a secondary binder in wet granulation tablet preparation either to granulate both soluble and insoluble APIs. This formulation will produce less hard tablets than that without MCC. The fast wicking action of MCC promotes rapid wetting of the powder mix. This is particularly useful in high moisture granulations as it binds the excess moisture and keeps the granules dry and free flowing.

4.5 MCC as disintegrant

Disintegrants expand and dissolve once it is in contact with water causing the tablet to break apart in the GI tract and release the active ingredients for absorption. It will break a tablet into smaller fragments therefore increasing the surface area of the active drug in the dosage form; hence it will also increase the rate of drug absorption. The mechanism of disintegrants in the tablet disintegration could be as either water uptake facilitators or tablet rupture promoters. MCC has been widely used as a disintegrant in dry compressions and wet granulation method for tablet manufacturing. It enhances drug dissolution by increasing the rate of tablet disintegration. Basically a disintegrant should provide the highest level of disintegration force at low use levels and utilizes dual disintegration mechanisms either in wicking or swelling for faster tablet disintegration.

The Avicel derivate showed the nature in a fast wicking rate of water with small elastic deformation. These properties provide the ability for tablet disintegration. However, Avicel has a tendency to develop static charges with increased moisture content. Sometimes it even can cause striation or separation in the granules. This occurs when the moisture content in Avicel is above 3%, in which the static charges during mixing and compression become more pronounced. The problem can be overcome by drying the Avicel prior the formulation process to reduce the moisture to lower level. Wet granulated Avicel will lose some of its disintegration properties when performing drying and compression during formulation [4]. In contrast with starch, it cannot be wet granulated without losing some of its disintegration properties. Normally, to overcome this problem, Avicel and starch are used in combination in order to facilitate effective and rapid disintegration of tablets.

MCC has a very high intraparticle porosity with approximately 90–95% of the surface area being internal [44]. Therefore the surface area is not directly influenced by the nominal particle size [58]. High porosity of MCC promotes swelling and disintegration of formulated tablets, which is attributed to either by the penetration of water into the hydrophilic tablet matrix by means of capillary action of the pores or even by a disruption of the hydrogen bonds. By increasing compaction pressure, water penetration into the tablets will decrease; therefore disintegration time will increase [54, 85].

In intramolecular view, water is only sorbed in the amorphous regions of MCC, which are more hydrophilic than the crystalline regions [3, 54]. Therefore the total amount of sorbed water is proportional to the fraction of amorphous material in the MCC crystallinity and is independent of the surface area [48]. The crystallinity of MCC determined by X-ray diffraction and infrared measurement was found to be in the range of 60–80% [53].

Recently, Avicel has been used as a disintegrant in orally disintegrating tablets. Besides being a disintegrant, it also acts as a dissolution enhancer. US Patent No 6350470 explains the use of Avicel as a disintegrating agent in effervescent drug delivery system for oral administration. In this system, by performing dry granulation, Avicel acts as disintegrant in a concentration of 5.20% [96]. Avicel acts as an effervescent penetration enhancer.

4.6 MCC as lubricant

Lubricants ensure that tablet formation and ejection can occur with low friction between the solid and die wall.

Avicel has an extremely low coefficient of friction, both static and dynamic, so that it has no lubricant requirement itself. However, when more than 20% of the drug and other excipients are added, lubrication is necessary.

4.7 MCC as glidant

In tablet formulation, glidant is used to promote powder flow by reducing interparticle friction and cohesion. Glidants can be used in combination with lubricants as they have no ability to reduce die wall friction. Normally, silica-based glidants like silicon dioxide, hydrated sodium silicoaluminate, silica hydrogel, etc. are used in tablet compression to promote good flow property. Proslov as a marketed product of coprocess excipient containing MCC is available which imparts superior flow, good compactibility, and dispersion to tablet formulation [97].

When used as excipient in direct compression, Prosolv SMCC® (JRS Pharma, Patterson, NY) can replace granulation step and significantly reduce excipient numbers and levels. Prosolv SMCC® formulations produce distinctive, uniform, and cost-effective tablets. It is available in three grades: Prosolv SMCC 50, Prosolv SMCC 90, and Prosolv SMCC HD 90. The products differ in average of particle size and bulk density [98]. They offer many benefits including enhanced mixing characteristics, enhanced flow properties, lower unit cost of production due to less excipients needed, and shorter disintegration time. Due to improvement in powder compactibility and dust-free handling during production, Prosolv facilitates less loss in production hence a higher manufacturing efficiency.

In a more recent study, it is reported that silicified MCC and MCC were found to be good plug formers in hard gelatin capsule shells. The study was conducted in a compaction simulator at tamping forces and piston speeds similar to those found in some filling machines. Several grades of silicified MCC and a particular grade of MCC having particle size of 90 μm produced plugs with a higher maximum breaking force than anhydrous lactose and Starch 1500 under similar compression conditions [99].

4.8 MCC as a spheronizing agent

MCC is an excipient of choice in a multiparticulate delivery of pellets prepared by extrusion spheronization. The extrusion-spheronization process aims to produce drugs into sphere-shaped tablets. Extrusion-spheronization process offers an alternative to traditional drug layering on pellets. This highly specialized process results in unique spherical, drug-loaded spherical pellets. Higher drug loading can be employed with this approach over that which looks impossible with conventional drug layering. The product, initially called as extrudates, is plastic without rigidity, which tends to agglomerate into very large spherical balls. The formulation mixture which will be manufactured by extrusion method must fulfill the requirements:

1. Cohesive and deformable in order to have good flow through the die without sticking and able to retain its shape after extrusion process

2. Plastic, so that it can proceed rolling process into spheres in the spheronizer but possesses non-cohesive property so that the final sphere form can remain discrete

MCC, especially Avicel PH-101, can act as an excellent extrusion-spheronization aid excipient that absorbs the water added to the formulation more as a molecular sponge. This ability alters the rheological properties of the wet mass, therefore enhancing the tensile strength of the wet mass during spheronization process through autoadhesion.

Avicel® PH-101 or Avicel PH-102 is highly recommended to be used for this method because it can reduce spheroid friability, prevent overwetting of spheres, and improve sphericity of pellets. Process sensitivity during the whole manufacture can be lessened to the lower level.

4.9 Sustained release applications

Recently, MCC has been widely used in the formulation of multiparticulate and matrix tablet dosage forms for sustained release drug delivery system. In general, hydrophilic polymers in matrix tablet formulation are included to form a viscous, gelling layer which can retard water penetration and acts as a barrier to drug release. Drug release is accomplished by diffusion through the gel layer and at the same time through erosion of this layer. Some studies proved that zero-order release profiles can be achieved by selection of appropriate polymers in addition of Avicel as fillers/binders.

5. Conclusions

Microcrystalline cellulose is a pure partially depolymerized cellulose synthesized from α-cellulose precursor with hydrolysis by mineral acids, usually in forms of a pulp from a fibrous plant. In the presence of water and acid, hydrolysis process breaks cellulose polymers into smaller chain polymers or microcrystals. Other celluloses, to which more soluble, such as beta and gamma celluloses, hemicelluloses and lignin are dissolved with acid and water, are separated out during washing. MCC is commonly dried from the slurry by spray-drying method. By varying spray-drying conditions, the degree of agglomeration and moisture content can be manipulated, in order to obtain particular particle sizes.

Mostly, a raw material for MMC is a cellulose pulp from fibrous plant such as conifer wood. Another source is from cotton either its linters, stalks, rags, fabric waste, or wool. Another study reported a potential source for MCC such as soybean, corn cob, water hyacinth, coconut shells, oil palm biomass residue, oil palm fronds, rice husk, sugar cane bagasse, jute, ramie, fibers and straw of flax, wheat straw, sorghum stalks, sisal fibers, mangosteen, alfa grass fibers, soybean hulls, orange mesocarp, Indian bamboo, roselle fiber, and alfa fiber. Seed flosses from milkweed pods, shrubs, and kapok (*Ceiba pentandra*) trees are also known as sources of cellulose.

A different manufacture will produce variability in properties of MCC due to the kinds of pulp used as raw materials and applied process parameters. This can be characterized from the physicochemical properties of product including moisture content, particle size, particle morphology, crystallinity, bulk density, and degree of polymerization.

Microcrystalline cellulose, according to many publications, is an excipient most widely used for direct compression. Besides, it also serves as a strong dry binder, tablet disintegrant, absorbent, filler or diluent, a lubricant, and anti-adherent.

Author details

Anis Yohana Chaerunisaa*, Sriwidodo Sriwidodo and Marline Abdassah
Department of Pharmaceutics and Pharmaceutical Technology, Faculty of Pharmacy, Padjadjaran University, Indonesia

*Address all correspondence to: anis.yohana.chaerunisaa@unpad.ac.id

References

[1] Carlin B. Direct compression and the role of filler-binders. In: Augsburger LL, Augsburger LL, Hoag SW, Hoag SW, editors. Pharmaceutical Dosage Forms: Tablets. 3rd edition. Vol. 2. Informa; 2008. pp. 173-216

[2] Shlieout G, Arnold K, Muller G. Powder and mechanical properties of microcrystalline cellulose with different degrees of polymerization. AAPS PharmSciTech. 2002;**3**:E11

[3] Suzuki T, Nakagami H. Effect of crystallinity of microcrystalline cellulose on the compactability and dissolution of tablets. European Journal of Pharmaceutics and Biopharmaceutics. 1999;**47**:225-230

[4] Landín M, Martínez-Pacheco R, Gómez-Amoza JL, Souto C, Concheiro A, Rowe RC. Effect of batch variation and source of pulp on the properties of microcrystalline cellulose. International Journal of Pharmaceutics. 1993;**91**:133-141

[5] Chauhan YP, Sapkal RS, Sapkal VS, Zamre GS. Microcrystalline cellulose from cotton rags (waste from garment and hosiery industries). International Journal of Chemical Sciences. 2009;**7**(2):681-688

[6] El-Sakhawy M, Hassan ML. Physical and mechanical properties of microcrystalline cellulose prepared from agricultural residues. Carbohydrate Polymers. 2007;**67**:1-10

[7] Chuayjuljit S, Su-uthai S, Charuchinda S. Poly(vinyl chloride) film filled with microcrystalline cellulose prepared from cotton fabric waste: Properties and biodegradability study. Waste Management & Research. 2010;**28**(2):109-117

[8] Rashid M, Gafur MA, Sharafat MK, Minami H, Miah MAJ, Ahmad H. Biocompatible microcrystalline cellulose particles from cotton wool and magnetization via a simple in situ co-precipitation method. Carbohydrate Polymers. 2017;**170**:72-79

[9] Uesu NY, Pineda EA, Hechenleitner AA. Microcrystalline cellulose from soybean husk: Effects of solvent treatments on its properties as acetylsalicylic acid carrier. International Journal of Pharmaceutics. 2000;**206**:85-96

[10] Suvachittanont S, Ratanapan P. Optimization of micro crystalline cellulose production from corn cob for pharmaceutical industry investment. Journal of Chemistry and Chemical Engineering. 2013;**7**:1136-1141

[11] Gaonkar SM, Kulkarni PR. Improved method for the preparation of microcrystalline cellulose from water hyacinth. Textile Dyer and Printer. 1987;**20**(26):19-22

[12] Gaonkar SM, Kulkarni PR. Microcrystalline cellulose from coconut shells. Acta Polymer. 1989;**40**:292-293

[13] Fahma F, Iwamoto S, Hori N, Iwata T, Takemura A. Isolation, preparation, and characterization of nanofibers from oil palm empty-fruit-bunch (OPEFB). Cellulose. 2010;**17**(5):977-985

[14] Mohamad Haafiz MK, Eichhorn SJ, Hassan A, Jawaid M. Isolation and characterization of microcrystalline cellulose from oil palm biomass residue. Carbohydrate Polymers. 2013;**93**(2):628-634

[15] Owolabia A, Haafiza M, Hossain M, Hussin H, Fazita N. Influence of alkaline hydrogen peroxide pre-hydrolysis on the isolation of microcrystalline cellulose from oil palm fronds. International Journal of Biological Macromolecules. 2017;**95**:1228-1234

[16] Ilindra A, Dhake JD. Microcrystalline cellulose from bagasse and rice straw. Indian Journal of Chemical Technology. 2008;**15**(5):497-499

[17] Paralikar KM, Bhatawdekar SP. Microcrystalline cellulose from bagasse pulp. Biological Wastes. 1988;**24**:75-77

[18] Padmadisastra Y, Gonda I. Preliminary studies of the development of a direct compression cellulose excipient from bagasse. Journal of Pharmaceutical Sciences. 1989;**78**(6):508-521

[19] Shah DA, Shah YD, Trivedi BM. Production of microcrystalline cellulose from sugar cane bagasse on pilot plant and its evaluation as pharmaceutical adjunct. Research and Industry. 1993;**38**(3):133-137

[20] Tang L-G, Hon DN-S, Pan S-H, Zhu Y-U, Wang Z, Wang Z-Z. Evaluation of microcrystalline cellulose. I. Changes in ultrastructural characteristics during preliminary acid hydrolysis. Journal of Applied Polymer Science. 1996;**59**:483-488

[21] Abdullah ABM. Production of jute microcrystalline cellulose. Journal of Bangladesh Academy of Science. 1991;**15**(2):85-87

[22] Jahan MS, Saeed A, He Z, Ni Y. Jute as raw material for the preparation of microcrystalline cellulose. Cellulose. 2011;**18**(2):451-459

[23] Kuga S, Brown RM. Lattice imaging of ramie cellulose. Polymer Communications Guildford. 1987;**28**(11):311-314

[24] Bochek AM, Shevchuk IL, Lavrentev VN. Fabrication of microcrystalline and powdered cellulose from short flax fiber and flax straw. Russian Journal of Applied Chemistry. 2003;**76**(10):1679-1682

[25] Monschein M, Reisinger C, Nidetzky B. Enzymatic hydrolysis of microcrystalline cellulose and pretreated wheat straw: A detailed comparison using convenient kinetic analysis. Bioresource Technology. 2013;**128**:679-687

[26] Ohwoavworhua FO, Adelakun TA. Non-wood fibre production of microcrystalline cellulose from *Sorghum caudatum*: Characterisation and tableting properties. Indian Journal of Pharmaceutical Science. 2010;**72**(3):295-301

[27] Bhimte NA, Tayade PT. Evaluation of microcrystalline cellulose prepared from sisal fibers as a tablet excipient: A technical note. Association of Pharmaceutical Scientists (AAPS). Pharmaceutical Science and Technology. 2007;**8**(1):E56-E62

[28] Winuprasith T, Suphantharika M. Microfibrillated cellulose from mangosteen (*Garcinia mangostana* L.) rind: Preparation, characterization, and evaluation as an emulsion stabilizer. Food Hydrocolloids. 2013;**32**(2):383-394

[29] Trache D, Donnot A, Khimeche K, Benelmir R, Brosse N. Physico-chemical properties and thermal stability of microcrystalline cellulose isolated from alfa fibres. Carbohydrate Polymers. 2014;**104**:223-230

[30] Trache D, Khimeche K, Mezroua A, Benziane M. Physicochemical properties of microcrystalline nitrocellulose from alfa grass fibers and its thermal stability. Journal of Thermal Analysis and Calorimetry. 2016;**124**(3):1485-1496

[31] Merci A, Urbano A, Grossmann MVE, Tischer CA, Mali S. Properties of microcrystalline cellulose extracted from soybean hulls by reactive

extrusion. Food Research International. 2015;**SI**(73):38-43

[32] Ejikeme PM. Investigation of the physicochemical properties of microcrystalline cellulose from agricultural wastes I: Orange mesocarp. Cellulose. 2008;**15**(1):141-147

[33] Ngozi UO, Chizoba NA, Ifeanyichukwu OS. Physico-chemical properties of microcrystalline cellulose derived from Indian Bamboo (*Bambusa vulgaris*). International Journal of Pharmaceutical Sciences Review and Research. 2014;**29**(2):5-9. Article No. 02

[34] Kiana LK, Jawaida M, Ariffina H, Alothmanb OY. Isolation and characterization of microcrystalline cellulose from roselle fibers. International Journal of Biological Macromolecules. 2017;**103**(2017):931-940

[35] Trachea D, Donnotb A, Khimechea K, Benelmirb R, Brosse N. Physico-chemical properties and thermal stability of microcrystalline cellulose isolated from Alfa fibres. Carbohydrate Polymers. 2014;**104**:223-230

[36] Hindi SSZ. Calotropis procera: The miracle shrub in the Arabian Peninsula. International Journal of Science and Engineering Investigations (IJSEI). 2013;**2**(16):48-57

[37] Thoorens G, Krier F, Leclercq B, Carlin B, Evrard B. Microcrystalline cellulose, a direct compression binder in a quality by design environment: A review. International Journal of Pharmaceutics. 2014;**473**(1-2):64-72

[38] Hindi SSZ, Abohassan RA. Cellulosic microfibril and its embedding matrix within plant cell wall. International Journal of Innovative Research in Science, Engineering and Technology. 2016;**5**(3):2727-2734

[39] Guy A. Cellulose, microcrystalline. In: Rowe RC, Sheskey PJ, Quinn ME, editors. Handbook of Pharmaceutical Excipients. Vol. 6. UK: Pharmaceutical Press; 2009. pp. 129-133, American Pharmacists Association (USA). ISBN 978 0 85369 792 3 (UK), ISBN 978 1 58212 135 2 (USA)

[40] Ohwoavworhua FO, Kunle OO, Ofoefule SI. Extraction and characterization of microcrystalline cellulose derived from *Luffa cylindrica* plant. African Journal of Pharmaceutical Research and Development. 2004;**1**:1-6

[41] Reier GE. Problem Solver. Avicel1 PH Microcrystalline Cellulose, NF, Ph Eur. JP, BP. 2000. Available from: http://www.fmcbiopolymer.com/Portals/bio/content/Docs/PS-Section% 2011.pdf

[42] Christiansen OB, Sardo MS. Find the optimum flash dryer to remove surface moisture. CEP magazine. 2001;54-58. Available from: http://www.barr-rosin.com/library_pdfs/find_optimum_flash_dryer_remove_moisture.pdf

[43] Albers J, Knop K, Kleinebudde P. Brand-to-brand and batch-to-batch uniformity of microcrystalline cellulose in direct tableting with a pneumo-hydraulic tablet press. La Pharmacie Industrielle. 2006;**68**:1420-1428

[44] Doelker E. Comparative compaction properties of various microcrystalline cellulose types and generic products. Drug Development and Industrial Pharmacy. 1993;**19**:2399-2471

[45] Landín M, Martínez-Pacheco R, Gómez-Amoza JL, Souto C, Concheiro A, Rowe RC. Influence of microcrystalline cellulose source and batch variation on the tabletting behaviour and stability of prednisone formulations. International Journal of Pharmaceutics. 26 April 1993;**91**(2-3):143-149

[46] Landín M, Martínez-Pacheco R, Gómez-Amoza JL, Souto C, Concheiro A, Rowe RC. Influence of Microcrystalline Cellulose Source and Batch Variation on the Tabletting. 1993

[47] Williams RO, Sriwongjanya M, Barron MK. Compaction properties of microcrystalline cellulose using tableting indices. Drug Development and Industrial Pharmacy. 1997;**23**:695-704

[48] Amidon GE, Houghton ME. The effect of moisture on the mechanical and powder flow properties of microcrystalline cellulose. Pharmaceutical Research. 1995;**12**:923-929

[49] Wu J-S, Ho H-O, Sheu M-T. A statistical design to evaluate the influence of manufacturing factors and material properties on the mechanical performances of microcrystalline cellulose. Powder Technology. 2001;**118**:219-228

[50] Wu J-S, Ho H-O, Sheu M-T. A statistical design to evaluate the influence of manufacturing factors on the material properties and functionalities of microcrystalline cellulose. European Journal of Pharmaceutical Sciences. 2001;**12**:417-425

[51] Reier GE. Fun facts about Avicel® microcrystalline cellulose also known as cellulose gel. 2013. Available from: http://www.fmcbiopolymer.com/Food/Home/News/FiftyYearsofAvicel.aspx

[52] Doelker E, Mordier D, Iten H, Humbert-Droz P. Comparative tableting properties of sixteen microcrystalline celluloses. Drug Development and Industrial Pharmacy. 1987;**13**:1847-1875

[53] Sun CC. Mechanism of moisture induced variations in true density and compaction properties of microcrystalline cellulose. International Journal of Pharmaceutics. 2008;**346**:93-101

[54] Bolhuis GK, Chowhan ZT. Materials for direct compaction. In: Alderborn G, Alderborn G, Nyström C, Nyström C, editors. Pharmaceutical Powder Compaction Technology. New York: Marcel Dekker, Inc.; 1996. pp. 419-500

[55] Nokhodchi A. An overview of the effect of moisture on compaction and compression. Pharmaceutical Technology. 2005;**46-66**

[56] Patel S, Kaushal AM, Bansal AK. Compression physics in the formulation development of tablets. Critical Reviews in Therapeutic Drug Carrier Systems. 2006;**23**:1-65

[57] Almaya A, Aburub A. Effect of particle size on compaction of materials with different deformation mechanisms with and without lubricants. AAPS PharmSciTech. 2008;**9**:414-418

[58] Gamble JF, Chiu WS, Tobyn M. Investigation into the impact of sub-populations of agglomerates on the particle size distribution and flow properties of conventional microcrystalline cellulose grades. Pharmaceutical Development and Technology. 2011;**16**:542-548

[59] Jivraj M, Martini LG, Thomson CM. An overview of the different excipients useful for the direct compression of tablets. Pharmaceutical Science & Technology Today. 2000;**3**:58-63

[60] Pesonen T, Paronen P. The effect of particle and powder properties on the mechanical properties of directly compressed cellulose tablets. Drug Development and Industrial Pharmacy. 1990;**16**:31-54

[61] Thoorens G, Krier F, Rozet E, Carlin B, Evrard B. Understanding the

impact of microcrystalline cellulose physicochemical properties on tabletability. International Journal of Pharmaceutics. 2015;**490**:47-54

[62] Hwang R-C, Peck GR. A systematic evaluation of the compression and tablet characteristics of various types of microcrystalline cellulose. Pharmaceutical Technology. June 2001:112-132

[63] Whiteman M, Yarwood RJ. Variations in the properties of microcrystalline cellulose from different sources. Powder Technology. 1988;**54**:71-74

[64] Herting MG, Kleinebudde P. Roll compaction/dry granulation: Effect of raw material particle size on granule and tablet properties. International Journal of Pharmaceutics. 2007;**338**:110-118

[65] Kushner J, Langdon BA, Hiller JI, Carlson GT. Examining the impact of excipient material property variation on drug product quality attributes: A quality-by-design study for a roller compacted, immediate release tablet. Journal of Pharmaceutical Sciences. 2011;**100**:2222-2239

[66] Kushner J. Utilizing quantitative certificate of analysis data to assess the amount of excipient lot-to-lot variability sampled during drug product development. Pharmaceutical Development and Technology. 2013;**18**:333-342

[67] Hasegawa M. Direct compression: Microcrystalline cellulose grade 12 versus classic grade 102. Pharmaceutical Technology. 2002;**26**:50-60. Available from: http://www.pharmtech.com/pharmtech/data/articlestandard//pharmtech/192002/18599/article.pdf

[68] Hlinak AJ, Kuriyan K, Morris KR, Reklaitis GV, Basu PK. Understanding critical material properties for solid dosage form design. Journal of Pharmaceutical Innovation. 2006;**1**:12-17

[69] Obae K, Iijima H, Imada K. Morphological effect of microcrystalline cellulose particles on tablet tensile strength. International Journal of Pharmaceutics. 1999;**182**:155-164

[70] Friedman R. Pharmaceutical quality systems: US perspective. Pharmaceutical Quality System (ICH Q10) Conference. 2011. Available from: http://www.fda.gov/downloads/drugs/ developmentapprovalprocess/manufacturing/ucm288108.pdf

[71] Vehovec T, Gartner A, Planinsek O, Obreza A. Influence of different types of commercially available microcrystalline cellulose on degradation of perindopril erbumine and enalapril maleate in binary mixtures. Acta Pharmaceutica. 2012;**62**:515-528

[72] Abdel-Hamid S, Alshihabi F, Betz G. Investigating the effect of particle size and shape on high speed tableting through radial die-wall pressure monitoring. International Journal of Pharmaceutics. 2011;**413**:29-35

[73] Liao Z, Zhang N, Zhao G, Zhang J, Liang X, Zhong S, et al. Multivariate analysis approach for correlations between material properties and tablet tensile strength of microcrystalline cellulose. Pharmazie. 2012;**67**:774-780

[74] Pönni R, Vuorinen T, Kontturi E. Proposed nano-scale coalescence of cellulose in chemical pulp fibers during technical treatments. BioResources. 2012;**7**:6077-6108

[75] Westermarck S, Juppo AM, Kervinen L, Yliruusi J. Microcrystalline cellulose and its microstructure in pharmaceutical processing. European Journal of Pharmaceutics and Biopharmaceutics. 1999;**48**:199-206

[76] Bolhuis GK, Armstrong NA. Excipients for direct compaction—An

update. Pharmaceutical Development and Technology. 2006;**11**:111-124

[77] Sheth BB, Bandelin FJ, Shangraw RF. Compressed tablets. In: Lachman L, Liberman HA, Schwartz JB, editors. Pharmaceutical Dosage Forms: Tablets. Vol. 2. New York, Basel, HongKong: Marcel Dekker Inc.; 1990. p. 109

[78] Schwartz JB, Lachman L. Compressed tablets by wet granulation. In: Bandelin JF, editor. Pharmaceutical Dosage Forms: Tablets. Vol. 1. New York, Basel, HongKong: Marcel Dekker Inc; 1990. p. 133

[79] Peck GE, Anderson NR, Banker GS. Principles of improved tablet production system design. In: Liebermann HA, Lachman L, Schwartz JB, editors. Pharmaceutical Dosage Forms: Tablets. Lea & Febiger; 1990. pp. 1-76

[80] Kása P, Bajdik J, Zsigmond Z, Pintye-Hódi K. Study of the compaction behaviour and compressibility of binary mixtures of some pharmaceutical excipients during direct compression. Chemical Engineering and Processing—Process Intensification. 2009;**48**:859-863

[81] Tho I, Bauer-Brandl A. Quality by design (QbD) approaches for the compression step of tableting. Expert Opinion on Drug Delivery. 2011;**8**:1631-1644

[82] Hentzschel CM, Sakmann A, Leopold CS. Comparison of traditional and novel tableting excipients: Physical and compaction properties. Pharmaceutical Development and Technology. 2012;**17**:649-653

[83] Ilic I, Govedarica B, Sibanc R, Dreu R, Srcic S. Deformation properties of pharmaceutical excipients determined using an in-die and out-die method. International Journal of Pharmaceutics. 2013;**446**:6-15

[84] Shi L, Chattoraj S, Sun CC. Reproducibility of flow properties of microcrystalline cellulose—Avicel PH102. Powder Technology. 2011;**212**:253-257

[85] Lahdenpää E, Niskanen M, Yliruusi J. Crushing strength, disintegration time and weight variation of tablets compressed from three Avicelä PH grades and their mixtures. European Journal of Pharmaceutics and Biopharmaceutics. 1997;**43**:315-322

[86] Wallace JW, Capozzi JT, Shangraw RF. Performance of pharmaceutical filler/binders as related to methods of powder characterization. Pharmaceutical Technology. 1983;7:94-104

[87] Patel NK, Upadhyay AH, Bergum JS, Reier GE. An evaluation of microcrystalline cellulose and lactose excipients using an instrumented single station tablet press. International Journal of Pharmaceutics. 1994;**110**:203-210

[88] Rubinstein MH. Tablets. In: Aulton ME, Aulton ME, editors. Pharmaceutics: The Science of Dosage Form Design. Churchill Livingstone; 1988

[89] Kushner J, Moore F. Scale-up model describing the impact of lubrication on tablet tensile strength. International Journal of Pharmaceutics. 2010;**399**:19-30

[90] Roberts RJ, Rowe RC. The effect of punch velocity on the compaction of a variety of materials. The Journal of Pharmacy and Pharmacology. 1985;**37**:377-384

[91] Ferrari F, Bertoni M, Bonferoni MC, Rossi S, Caramella C, Nyström C. Investigation on bonding and disintegration properties of pharmaceutical materials. International Journal of Pharmaceutics. 1996;**136**:71-79

[92] Saigal N, Baboota S, Ahuja A, Ali J. Microcrystalline cellulose as a versatile excipient in drug research. Journal of Young Pharmacists. 2009;**1**:6-12

[93] Bala R, Khanna S, Pawar PK. Formulation and optimization of fast dissolving intraoral drug delivery system for clobazam using response surface methodology. Journal of Advanced Pharmaceutical Technology & Research. 2013;**4**:151-159

[94] Mostafa HF, Ibrahim MA, Sakr A. Development and optimization of dextromethorphan hydrobromide oral disintegrating tablets: Effect of formulation and process variables. Pharmaceutical Development and Technology. 2013;**18**:454-463

[95] Saha S, Sahiwala AF. Multifunctional coprocessed excipients for improved tabletting performance. Expert Opinion on Drug Delivery. 2009;**6**:197-208

[96] Indiran PS, Robinson JR, Eichman JD, Khankari RK, Hontz J, Gupte SV. Effervescent drug delivery system for oral administration. US 6350470. 2002

[97] Rios M. Debating Excipient Functionality. Special Report. International Pharmaceutical Excipients Council. 2006. Available from: http://ipecamericas.org/newsletters/PT9-30-06e.pdf [Accessed: Mar 19, 2009]

[98] Ausburger LL. Hard Shell Capsules. FMC Biopolymer. 2008. Available from: http://www.fmcbiopolymer.com/Portals/bio/content/Docs/Pharmaceuticals/Problem%20Solver/8_hardshellcapsules.pdf [Accessed: Mar 25, 2009]

[99] Guo M, Muller FX, Augsburger LL. Evaluation of the plug formation process of silicified microcrystalline cellulose. International Journal of Pharmaceutics. 2002;**233**:99-109

Section 2

Estimation of Bioavailability

Chapter 4

Bioavailability and Bioequivalence Studies

Divvela Hema Nagadurga

Abstract

In vivo bioavailability studies are performed for new drug to establish essential pharmacokinetic parameters including rate of absorption, extent of absorption, rates of excretion and metabolism and elimination half-life after a single and multiple dose administration. These essential pharmacokinetic parameters are useful in establishing dosage regimens. Bioequivalence used to assess the expected *in vivo* biological equivalence of two proprietary preparations of drug products. If two drugs are bioequivalent, it means that they are expected to be same for all intents and purposes. In determining bioequivalence between two drugs such as a reference drug or brand and potential to be test drug or marketed generic drug. Pharmacokinetic studies are conducted whereby each of the drugs is administered in a cross over study to healthy volunteer's subjects. Plasma is obtained at regular intervals and assayed for parent drug or metabolite concentration to compare the two drugs. For comparison purpose of two formulations, the plasma concentration data are used to assess key pharmacokinetic parameters. If 90% confidence interval for the ratio of the geometric least square means of peak plasma concentration, area under curve of test and reference drugs are within 80–125%, then bioequivalence will be established.

Keywords: bioavailability, bioequivalence studies, pharmacokinetic parameters, cross over study, area under curve

1. Introduction

Bioavailability is defined as relative amount of drug from an administered dosage which enters the systemic circulation and the rate at which the drug appears in the systemic circulation. The bioavailability studies are done by measuring the concentration of the drug in the plasma or blood after administration of drug following systemic protocol of studies and documented over time. The systemic protocol is helpful for clinical trials in the early drug development, and the data obtained are used in subsequent bioequivalence studies. Bioequivalence studies were carried out to distinguish between two pharmaceutical products containing the same active substance. One drug formulated into two different formulations if they show to be therapeutically equivalent to one another in order to be considered interchangeable.

Pharmacokinetics of drug deals with the change in drug concentration in plasma and/or its metabolites in the human or animal body with respect to time following administration of the pharmaceutical product. Bioequivalence studies are used to assess the expected *in vivo* biological equivalence of two proprietary preparations of a drug. If two pharmaceutical products are said to be bioequivalent, then they would be expected to be the same for all intents and purposes. Bioequivalence of a drug product is achieved if its extent and rate of absorption are not statically significantly different from those of reference product when administered at the same molar dose. If the bioavailability of two formulations administered in the same molar dose is similar, then they are said to be bioequivalent [1–10]. Different test methods are available to assess equivalence, including:

1. Comparative bioavailability studies, in which the active drug substance is measured in an accessible biological fluid such as plasma

2. Comparative clinical trials

3. Comparative pharmacodynamic studies in humans

Bioavailability and bioequivalence studies are required to ensure therapeutic equivalence between a pharmaceutically equivalent test drug and a generic drug or reference drug. Ensuring uniformity in standards of quality, efficacy, and safety of pharmaceutical products is the fundamental responsibility of central drugs standard control organization (CDSCO) [11]. Bioequivalence has to be considered for various products containing active ingredients marketed under different licensees are clinically equivalent and interchangeable. Submission of application for new drugs under schedule Y should be required to furnish the bioavailability and bioequivalence data, that is, mainly focus on the drug release from the pharmaceutical dosage form and subsequent absorption into the systemic circulation.

Comparative bioavailability or relative bioavailability refers to a comparison of two pharmaceutical dosage forms in terms of their relative rate and extent of absorption. In some cases, two pharmaceutical formulations exhibit markedly different bioavailability, for example, a rapidly absorbed elixir and more slowly absorbed capsule. In other cases, two different dosage formulations such as tablet and a capsule may or may not exhibit very similar bioavailability [12].

$$\text{Comparative bioavailability} = \frac{AUCpo \times Doseiv}{AUCiv \times Dosepo}. \tag{1}$$

Absolute bioavailability refers to an active pharmaceutical ingredient reaching the systemic circulation and fraction of drug absorbed ranges from 0 to 1. If F is zero, it means no drug absorptions, and the drug is completely absorbed in the systemic circulation if F = 1. The total amount of drug reaching the systemic circulation is directly proportional to the area under curve (AUC), and fraction of drug absorbed is determined by comparing the respective AUCs of the test product and the same dose of the drug administered intravenously [13].

$$\text{Absolute bioavailability} = \frac{AUCpo}{AUCiv} \tag{2}$$

1.1 Types of studies required in bioequivalence studies

For certain drugs, *in vivo* equivalence was done through either a bioequivalence study or a comparative clinical pharmacodynamic study. For oral immediate drug release formulations with systemic action have one or more adverse conditions like narrow therapeutic window, steep dose-response curve, nonlinear pharmacokinetics, presystemic elimination, unfavorable physicochemical properties.

Physicochemical properties such as solubility and instability of the drug, metastable transformation, poor permeability, etc., are bioavailability problems related to the drug or drugs having similar chemical structure or formulations, where a high ratio of excipients to active ingredients exists. Drugs administered other than oral and parenteral formulations design act by systemic absorption, sustained release drug formulations design act by systemic absorption, fixed dose combination products with systemic action, nonsolution pharmaceutical products which are for nonsystemic use and intended act without systemic absorption are also studied.

In these cases, the bioequivalence concept is not suitable, and then comparative clinical or pharmacodynamic studies are required for proving equivalence. Bioequivalence studies are used to establish links between the early and late clinical trial formulations, formulations used in clinical trials and stability studies, clinical trial formulations and to be marketed drug products. In each comparison, the new formulation or new method of manufacture shall be the test drug, and the prior formulation shall be considered as the reference drug.

1.2 When no need of bioequivalence studies

In some formulations, bioequivalence studies are not required if bioequivalence between a test drug and a reference drug may be considered self-evident with no further requirement for documentation such as when a gas is in the form of test drug, when test drugs are to be administered parenterally such as subcutaneous, intramuscular, intravenous, etc. as aqueous solution and contain the same drug in the same concentration and the same excipients in comparable concentrations. Bioequivalence studies are not required for when the test drug is in the form of solution for oral use and contains the drug in the same dose and does not contain an excipient that is known to affect gastro-intestinal absorption of the drug; when the test drug is in the form of an ophthalmic or topical product prepared as aqueous solution and contains the same active ingredients in the same concentrations and essentially the same excipients in comparable concentrations when the test drug is in the form of powder for reconstitution as a solution and the solution meets either above second and third points, when a test drug is in the form of an inhalation or a nasal spray tested by administered with or without the same device used for reference drug.

2. Design and conduct of pharmacokinetic studies

2.1 Study object

The object of the bioavailability study decides the study protocol. A study protocol used for estimating pharmacokinetic parameters is different from a bioequivalence study carried out for comparing the test formulation with standard formulation.

2.2 Study design

The main object of the experimental design is to minimize the experimental variables and to avoid a bias [14]. *In vivo* bioavailability study is determined by taking into consideration of the following points:

1. The nature of the reference drug and the dosage form to be tested

2. Benefit risk ratio considerations in regard to testing in humans

3. The availability of analytical methods

4. What is the scientific questions to be answered

Bioavailability studies are influenced by various factors such as age, sex, disease state, food habits, physical and mental health condition, body weight human volunteer, experimental design, time of administration, time of sampling, analytical method used and compartment model used in estimating pharmacokinetic parameters or bioavailability that contribute to the observed blood concentration time profile. Therefore, it is necessary to consider all these important factors in a study design.

The bioavailability study should be designed in such a way that the formulation effect can be distinguished from other effects. If two formulations are to be compared, a two-period, two-sequence crossover design is the design of choice which should ideally be equal to or more than five half-lives that have to be measured. Alternative study designs include the parallel design for very long half-life substances with highly variable disposition [15].

In the following sections, various factors are discussed keeping the bioequivalence study also in mind. However, they are valid for simple bioavailability studies also.

2.2.1 Parallel design

In a parallel design, two formulations are administered to two groups of volunteers. To avoid a bias, formulations may be administered randomly to the volunteers. The major disadvantage of this design is that the intersubject variation is not being corrected. It has been proved beyond doubt that most of the times intersubject variation is greater than the variation between any formulation. Therefore, a cross over design is preferred in bioavailability or bioequivalence trails to avoid influence of a intersubject variation. This design is used mainly for drug, and its metabolites have long elimination half-life. The carryover effects or dropouts were less in parallel studies compared to crossover studies.

2.2.2 Crossover design

As recommended by the USFDA [7], in most bioequivalence studies, a test drug is compared with the standard reference drug in a group of normal healthy subjects of age 18–55 years, each receives both the treatments alternately, in a crossover fashion (two-period, two-treatment crossover design), with the two phases of treatment separated by a washout period of generally a week's duration and it mainly depends on the half-life of the drug [16]. If elimination half-life of the drug increases, the washout period also increases. The drug formulation either test or reference is given to each human volunteer randomly but an equal number of subjects receives each treatment in each period, as given in **Table 1**. In case of two treatments, groups 1 and 2, one group receives the treatment in the order A and B, and the second group receives in the reverse order B and A. A similar allocation is done in case of a three-treatment crossover design (three-period, three-treatment crossover design). Intersubject variability is observed for several drugs in clearance. The intrasubject coefficient of variation (approximately 15%) is usually substantially smaller than that between subjects (approximately 30%), and therefore crossover designs are generally recommended for bioequivalence studies.

In crossover design, the treatments are compared on the same human subject, and the intersubject variability is reduced. Both the designs depend on the three fundamental statistical concepts of study design, and these are randomization, replication, and error control. Randomization means allocation of treatments to the

Group No.	Subject in group	Treatment for period No.			
Two-way crossover					
		I	II		
1.	1, 2, 3, 4, 5, 6	A	B		
2.	7, 8, 9, 10, 11, 12	B	A		
Three-way crossover					
		I	II	III	
1.	1, 2, 3, 4, 5, 6	A	C	B	
2.	7, 8, 9, 10, 11, 12	B	A	C	
3.	13, 14, 15, 16, 17, 18	C	B	A	
Four-way crossover					
		I	II	III	IV
1.	1, 2, 3, 4, 5, 6	A	B	C	D
2.	7, 8, 9, 10, 11, 12	B	D	A	C
3.	13, 14, 15, 16, 17, 18	C	A	D	B
4.	19, 20, 21, 22, 23, 24	D	C	B	A

Table 1.
Latin square design.

subjects without bias. Replication involves the application of more than one experimental subject for reliable estimates than a single observation and also provides a more precise measurement of treatment effects. The number of replicates required mainly depends upon the degree of differences to be detected and inherent variability of the data. Commonly used cross over designs in bioavailability trails are Latin square cross over design and balanced incomplete block design.

A standard approach for conducting a comparative bioavailability study to use a randomized, balanced, cross over design called Latin square or complete cross over design is as shown in **Table 1**. Incomplete block design (BIBD) eliminates many of the difficulties encountered with the Latin square design. In this, each subject receives not more than two formulations, each formulation is administered the same number of times and each pair of formulations occurs together in the same number of subjects. **Table 2** shows BIBD four formulations A, B, C, and D. In this design, as discussed above, each subject receives two formulations, each formulation is administered six times and each pair of formulations occurs together in two subjects (the pairs are AB, AC, AD, BC, BD, and CD).

2.3 Washout period

In a Latin square cross over design, each subject receives each formulation, and even in BIBD, each subject receives two formulations at different occasions. The time interval between the two treatments is called "washout period." Washout period is required for the elimination of the administered dose of a drug so as to avoid the carryover. For most of drugs in crossover design, at least 10 half-lives should be allowed between treatments. This should ensure an elimination of 99.9% of the administered dose and a maximum carryover of less than 0.1% from first treatment. The number of washout period is a function of the half-life and the dose of the drug administered. The number of washout periods in a study depends upon the type of crossover design used and the number of formulations to be evaluated.

Subject	Treatment for period No.	
	I	II
1	A	B
2	B	A
3	A	C
4	C	A
5	A	D
6	D	A
7	B	C
8	C	B
9	B	D
10	D	B
11	C	D
12	D	C

Table 2.
Balanced incomplete block design (BIBD) for four formulations.

In case of digitoxin, which has a half-life of 6–9 days, the total study period exceeds 1 year if four formulations have to be evaluated using Latin square design. Because a very large number of drugs have been found to have half-lives between 1 and 10 hours, a washout period of 1 week was usually found suitable in most of the reported studies. It should be noted that the metabolites of the drug should also be eliminated from the body before the commencement of next treatment.

2.4 Drug product and reference standard

Test product may be new drug formulations developed by pharmaceutical technologists or new dosage forms of an existing drug. A test product may be compared to a reference standard recognized by the Food and Drug Administration for getting approval for marketing the drug product. Test product are generally evaluated to select best dosage form of a new drug or existing drug among different dosage forms, to select the best formulation of a new drug or existing drug among different formulations that have shown equal performance *in vitro* tests and to compare biological performance of a test product to that of a recognized standard [17, 18].

A generic product has to compare with some standard dosage form to verify it's *in vivo* performance. In general, Food and Drug Administration (FDA) accepts any innovator's drug product as a reference standard. The innovator is the one who originally received approval from the FDA to market the product in the country. Sometime, several manufactures may hold approval for certain drugs. Therefore, any one of the permitted drug products can be used as a reference standard. In many of these instances, the FDA would request that only of these products be used as a reference product in order to obtain a more easily comparable data.

Most of the times orally administered dosage forms are subjected for bioavailability studies. However, dosage forms administered by other routes such as buccal, transdermal, and intramuscular should also be evaluated for their biological performance. The therapeutic utility of these dosage forms depends on the rate and extent of absorption of the drug from these dosage forms. Orally administered dosage forms show a much variation in their performance because of intersubject and intrasubject variations.

2.5 Single versus multiple dose study design

If the dosage forms are to be evaluated only for bioequivalence purposes, single dose studies are sufficient. This is because the relative bioavailability of most tablets and capsules can be determined on a single dose basis and usually this is predictive of multiple dose levels. Dosage forms determined for a single dose administration for a therapeutic benefit such as analgesic for the relief of head ache needs only single dose studies [19]. However, certain dosage forms designed to achieve special release profiles of drugs may require multiple dose studies like time release products, enteric-coated preparations, and some intramuscular injections. Even the drugs that undergo the first pass metabolism do need a multiple dose study.

2.6 Administration of drug products and sampling

Administration of drug products or formulations to the subjects should be based on randomization. After the administration, blood samples are withdrawn from the subjects at fixed time intervals. Some time is taken to withdraw a sample from each subject, and the total time difference between first subject and the last subject may range from 10 to 20 minutes depending upon the number of subjects and technicians involved in the study. If the sampling schedule is not followed rigorously in the same sequential manner, significant differences can conceivably exist in the actual duration of the drug in the body and the stated sampling time given for each subject. This 10 to 20 min difference in sample withdrawal from each subject during the study would represent a substantial change in the drug concentrations observed in the blood if under these conditions treatments are administered to the subjects in a sequential manner [20, 21].

If the bioavailability of a given dosage form is to be evaluated by a blood level study, some estimate of the area under the serum concentration versus time curve, peak plasma concentration (C_{max}), and time of peak plasma concentration (T_{max}) must be obtained from the study. Therefore, the frequency of sampling and the duration of sampling are very important for study. It will vary with the drug. There must be sufficient sampling points to allow for proper evaluation of the area under the blood level curve. A blood sampling done up to three to five half-lives of the drug, and if the half-life of the drug is not known, blood sampling should proceed until 1/10 or 1/20 of the peak levels are reached.

Urinary excretion studies are used when it is either not possible to measure a given drug in the blood, plasma or serum or when ethical considerations do not allow the collection of samples over a period of time. The advantage of this method is it involves noninvasive method of sampling, concentration of the drug in the urine is often greater than serum and the amount of the drug excreted in urine is obtained directly. But it is not useful in estimating the absorption rate of rapidly absorbed drugs and sometimes metabolites may interfere with the estimation of the unchanged drug in the urine sample.

Sampling must be continued for a sufficient time period to ensure that the area extrapolated from the time of the last measured concentration to infinite time should be less than 20% of the total AUC. AUC calculations are not useful in case of enterohepatic recycling where the terminal elimination rate constant cannot be calculated accurately. In such case, at least three sampling points from absorption phase, three to four points from Tmax and four points during the elimination phase has been taken. Intervals between successive sampling points in terminal elimination phase are used to calculate the elimination rate constant. It should not be longer than the half-life of the study drug.

2.7 Selection of the number of subjects

The number of subjects should be sufficient in the study to allow for possible withdrawals or dropouts. In initial study, it is acceptable to replace a subject withdrawal or dropout once it has provided the substituted subject follows the same protocol originally intended for the withdrawn subject and subject is tested under similar conditions. The number of subjects involved in a study is determined by the following considerations:

1. The level of significant should be 0.05

2. The error variance associated with the primary characteristics to be studied as estimated from a pilot experiment, from previous studies

3. The expected deviation from the reference drug compatible with bioequivalence

4. The required power, normally >80% to detect the maximum allowable difference in primary characteristics to be studied

2.7.1 Selection criteria for subjects

The studies should be performed on healthy adult volunteers with the aim to minimize variability between the study drugs. Subjects may be males or females; however, the choice of gender should be consistent with usage and safety criteria of the drug. To minimize intra and intersubject variation, the study design should be standardized as much as possible and acceptable.

2.7.2 Fasting and fed state considerations

Generally, a single dose study should be conducted after an overnight fast (at least 10 hours) and subsequent fasting of 4 hours after administration dosing. For multiple dose studies, 2 hours of fasting before and after the dose are acceptable. Estimation of C_{max} and T_{max} for the modified release products or drug is given with food in such case fed state studies also been carried out in addition to the normal fasting state bioavailability studies [22]. During fed state studies, the consumption of a high fat breakfast of 950–1000 KCals is required before dosing. The food intake containing at least 50% of these calories must come from fat, 15–20% calories from proteins, and the remaining from carbohydrates. A single standard diet should be followed taking into consideration of all the Indian subcontinent people. The high fat breakfast must be consumed approximately 15 minutes before dosing in fed state condition.

2.8 Study conditions

Study conditions such as study environment, diet, fluid intake, post dosing postures, exercise, sampling schedules, etc. are monitored during studies. These conditions are stated in the protocol, and at the end of the study, these should be complied, to assure that all variability factors involved in the study to minimize the products to be tested. Least 48 hours before commencement, the study subjects abstain from smoking, drinking alcohol, xanthine containing foods, coffee, tea and beverages, and fruit juices.

2.9 Steady state studies

Steady state study is considered in the following conditions:

1. The drug has a long terminal elimination half-life

2. Blood concentrations after a single dose cannot be achieved for a sufficient time.

3. For drugs, which are toxic or have adverse effects that are ethically should not be administered to patients but they are a necessary part of therapy (cytotoxics).

4. For modified release products or sustained release products which assess the fluctuation in plasma drug concentration at steady state.

5. Where the drug is likely to accumulate in the body.

6. For drugs that exhibit nonlinear, that is, dose or time dependent pharmacokinetics.

7. For combination products where the ratio of plasma concentration of the individual drugs is important.

8. For those drug which induce their own metabolism

9. For enteric coated preparations where the coating is innovative.

2.10 Analysis of biological samples

Ideally, the biological samples collected as per the sampling procedure have to be analyzed immediately after the study but most of the times the samples are stored for several days before subjected to analysis. During storage, the drug may undergo a chemical degradation, adsorption on the walls of the container, etc., so storage of plasma samples is an important aspect of bioavailability studies. The analytical method used for the estimation of the active ingredient responsible for the therapeutic efficacy must be selective and sensitive. Drugs, that undergo the first pass effect exhibit different unchanged drug/metabolite ratio depending on the rate of absorption. In the analysis of blood and urine, the major problem is to extract quantitatively and then separate the intact drug from its major metabolites or even to separate a mixture of two or more drugs from their metabolite.

2.11 Methods of assessment of bioavailability

Pharmacokinetic methods are used for the assessment of bioavailability of drug products that exists as a linear relation between the drug level in the biological fluid and therapeutic response. Therefore, these methods are also known indirect methods. Because therapeutically active drug can be accurately measured in biological fluids, plasma and urine data give the most objective information on bioavailability [23].

2.11.1 Indirect methods or pharmacokinetic methods

Plasma data are most widely used and accepted method for the assessment of bioavailability of the drug product. The basic assumption in this method is that drug products that are bioequivalent product super imposable plasma level time curve. The parameters T_{max} and C_{max} are the measures of the rate of absorption of the drug, while the parameters AUC is a measure of the extent of absorption.

Urinary excretion method is based on the general observation that the rate of urinary excretion of a drug is directly proportional to the concentration of the drug in the blood. Therefore, the bioavailability can be calculated as the ratio of the total amount of the unchanged drug recovered in urine following the administration of test and standard formulations. Urinary metabolite excretion data are not used for the estimation of bioavailability since the drug can undergo metabolism at different sites including the gut and liver, and the rates of metabolism may vary because of various reasons.

The relative bioavailability should lie within an acceptance range of 0.80–1.25 if 90% confidence interval is considered. In case of an especially narrow therapeutic range, the acceptance range may need to be tighter. In rare cases such as highly variable drugs, a wider acceptance range may be acceptable if it has right clinical justification. C_{max} ratio is the measure of relative bioavailability that may be more variable than the AUC ratio, and a wider acceptance range may be acceptable. The range used in the protocol should be justified taking into account safety and efficacy consideration. Tmax is a measure of release or action or signs for a relation to adverse effects.

2.11.2 Direct methods or pharmacodynamic methods

The pharmacodynamic methods are used when assessment of bioavailability by pharmacokinetic methods is not possible due to nonavailability of a sensitive analytical method for the measurement of the drug or the analytical methods lacks sufficient accuracy and/or reproducibility. The two pharmacodynamic methods used for the estimation of bioavailability are based on the measurement of acute pharmacological effect and clinical response. In order to estimate the bioavailability of a drug product accurately by measurement of acute pharmacological effect, the following criteria should meet. These are an easily measurable response such as heart rate, ECG, blood pressure, pupil diameter, etc. and an established dose-related response curve.

2.12 Statistical analysis of the data and analysis of variance (ANOVA)

Due to biological and experimental variations, some differences always exist, and it is necessary to ascertain whether these differences are simply chance occurrences or are due to actual differences in treatment administered to the subjects. Statistical methods are used to evaluate the pharmacokinetic data in order to identify the different sources of variation and if possible to measure the contribution of each identified variable and isolate the specific observation of primary interest. The analysis of variance (ANOVA), a statistical procedure that used for a crossover design is widely used method in bioavilability testing [24].

The pharmacokinetic parameters derived from blood drug concentration and time from bioavailability studies are subjected to ANOVA. In ANOVA, the variance is due to subjects, periods, and treatment. The classical null hypothesis test is considered where H0: $\mu T = \mu R$ if the pharmaceutical products are bioequivalent and alternate hypothesis therefore is H1: $\mu T \neq \mu R$ where products are bioinequivalent where μT and μR are the expected mean bioavailability of the test and reference or standard drug, respectively.

Bioavailability studies are designed in two ways, and these are design 1 and design 2. Design 1 is parallel design in which the subjects divide into two treatment groups and assign one treatment to each group. Design 2 is crossover design in which each subject has one block and applies both the treatments to each subject with washout period in between them. In a parallel design, variability due to the treatment is considered, and in the crossover design, variability due to treatment, subject, and period are considered to minimize variability. Error sum of squares in design 1 (SSE1) and sum of error sum of squares in design 2 (SSE2) are equal. The error mean sum of square for design 1 (MSE1) will be greater than the error mean sum of square for design 2 (MSE2) if the degrees of freedom for SSE are the same in the both designs then error variability is greater in the parallel group design compared to the crossover design (**Tables 3** and **4**).

The mean sum of squares is compared with the mean sum of squares due to error (F = MST/MSE), and if these are comparable, no difference between the levels of a factor is concluded, otherwise a difference is achieved. The treatment mean sum of squares is larger than the error mean sum of squares if difference is achieved between the treatments. Then the chances of getting treatment mean sum of squares being bigger than the error mean sum of squares are more in design 2 compared to design 1. Therefore, chances of showing a statistically significant difference are higher in design 2 compared to design 1. This is equivalent to saying that design 2 is more competent than design 1. Null hypothesis H0 μT = μR provides an assessment amount of drug absorbed from the test product is identical or equal or similar to the amount of drug absorbed from the reference. They may be different or nearly equal but not identical in most of the cases. If the trial is run under tightly controlled conditions and the number of subjects is large enough, no matter how small the difference between the formulations and it will be detected as significant. The difference may give rise to following anomalies due to a large difference between two formulations, sample size not large enough (**Table 5**).

In some cases, simple null hypothesis was inappropriate and alternative approach to ANOVA for bioequivalence studies is considered as Type I and II error. Type I error is a manufacturer's risk that is explained by probability of rejecting a formulation which is in fact bioequivalent. Manufacturer's risk is the probability (α = 0.05) of rejecting H0 when H0 is true. Similarly, type II error is the consumer's risk that is explained as the probability (β) of accepting a formulation which is bioinequivalent that is accepting H0 when H0 is false. FDA restricts the power of the test which should be 80% and the consumer's risk β to 20%, but this may not a satisfactory solution for either the consumer or the regulatory agencies. It makes

Sources of variance	Degree of freedom (D F)	Sum of squares (SS)	Mean of squares (MS)	F statistic
Treatment	T-1	SST	MST	MST/MSE
Subjects	N-1	SSS	MSS	MSS/MSE
Period	T-1	SSP	MSP	MSP/MSE
Error	(T-1)(N-2)	SSE	MSE	
Total	Tn-1			

T is the number of treatments, SST-sum of squares due to treatments, SSP-sum of squares due to period, MSS-mean sum of squares due to subjects, MST-mean sum of squares due to treatments, MSP-mean sum of squares due to period, and N is the number of subjects.

Table 3.
Analysis of variance (ANOVA) table for t-period, t-treatment crossover design.

Sources of variations	Sum of squares (SS)	Degree of freedom (DF)	Mean sum of squares (MSS)	F statistic
Between treatments	SST1	1	MST1	MST1/ MSE1
Error	SSE1	N-2	MSE1	
Total		N-1		

Table 4.
Design 1 A comparison of ANOVA for parallel group design and 2-treatment, 2-period crossover design with n subjects.

Sources of variance	Degree of freedom (DF)	Sum of squares (SS)	Mean of squares (MS)	F statistic
Between Treatments	1	SST2	MST2	MST2/MSE2
Subjects	N-1	SSS2	MSS2	
Between Period	1	SSP2	MSP2	
Errors	N-2	SSE2	MSE2	
Total	2N-1			

Table 5.
Design 2A comparison of ANOVA for parallel group design and 2-treatment, 2-period crossover design with n subjects.

sense that the regulatory authorities should control the consumer's risk and let the pharmaceutical company decide how much manufacturer's risk they are willing to accept. According to FDA guidelines for bioavailability studies state that "Products whose rate and extent of absorption differ by 20% or less are generally bioequivalent." The main object of bioequivalence studies is not in testing the null hypothesis of equality but to assess the difference between in two treatments groups and bioequivalence studies of two formulations is concluded that the difference is within 20% of the reference mean.

2.13 Characteristics to be investigated during bioequivalence studies

Evaluation of bioavailability and bioequivalence studies will be based upon the measurement of concentrations of the active drug substances in the plasma with respective of time. In some situations, the measurements of an active or inactive metabolite may be necessary. These situations include where the concentrations of the drugs may be too low to accurately measure in the biological matrix, limitations of the analytical method, unstable drugs, and drugs with a very short half-life. Racemates should be measured by an achiral assay method. Measurement of individual enantiomers in bioequivalence studies is required where they exhibit different primary efficacy, safety activity, pharmacodynamic and pharmacokinetic characteristics with the minor enantiomer. The pharmacokinetic parameters for product are C_{max}, T_{max}, $AUC_{0\text{-}t}$, and $AUC_{0\text{-}\infty}$ and for steady state are $AUC_{0\text{-}\tau}$, C_{max}, C_{min}, and degree of fluctuation should be calculated from the plasma time concentration profile.

2.14 Bioavailability and bioequivalence testing

Bioavailability and bioequivalence testing are carried out for two formulations such as new and commercially marketed brand drug [25]. These studies are conducted by experimental designs such as parallel and cross over design in healthy volunteer subjects but occasionally in patients. After administration of formulation under standard study conditions, plasma samples are withdrawn at regular time intervals and assayed for parent drug or occasionally metabolite concentration in plasma or urine. In some cases, concentration of drug in the blood is neither feasible nor possible to compare. Plasma concentration data are used to determine the pharmacokinetic parameters such as AUC, C_{max}, T_{max}, and absorption lag time (T_{lag}). Bioavailability studies should be conducted at different doses, especially when the drug follows nonlinear pharmacokinetics. In addition to a data from bioequivalence studies, other data may need to be submitted for evidence to meet regulatory requirements for bioequivalence includes analytical method validation and *in vitro-in vivo* correlation studies.

2.15 Criteria for bioequivalence

A 90% confidence interval is considered to establish bioequivalence for AUC, T_{max}, and C_{max} which should fall within the range of 80–125%. A 5% level of significance is taken for rejection of one sided t-test with the null hypothesis of bioequivalence. In bioavailability studies, closer limits are considered for drug that have a narrow therapeutic index, serious dose-related toxicity, steep dose, effect curve, and nonlinear pharmacokinetics within the therapeutic dose range. A wider acceptance range may be admissible if it is based on sound clinical justification. In case of suprabioavailability, a reformulation of the drug product is required and again bioequivalence study has to be carried out. Application of new formulation is required to support the clinical trial data especially for dosage recommendations. Such formulations are usually not being accepted as therapeutically equivalent to the existing reference drug.

3. Regulatory definitions

3.1 Australia

The Therapeutics Goods Administration (TGA) considers two formulations to be bioequivalent if the ratios between the two formulations of C_{max} and AUC should lie in the range of 0.80–1.25 and T_{max} should also be similar between the two formulations [25]. There are closer limits for drugs with a narrow therapeutic index and saturable metabolism. Thus, no generic drug formulations exist in for digoxin or phenytoin for instance in the Australian market.

3.2 Europe

European Economic Area considers two formulations to be bioequivalent if they have pharmaceutically equivalency and their bioavailabilities are similar after administration in the same molar dose with respect to both efficacy and safety. For bioequivalence of two dosage forms, 90% confidence intervals are considered as Australia.

3.3 United States

In case of FDA, two formulations are bioequivalent if the 90% confidence interval of the relative mean of C_{max}, $AUC_{0\text{-}t}$, and $AUC_{0\text{-}\infty}$ of the test or generic formulation should be within 80–125% in the fasting state. Sometimes, fed state bioequivalent comparison studies were carried out for test to reference formulations where required to administer the formulations after an appropriate meal at a specified time before taking the drug to know the food effect. Food effect study requires the same statistical evaluation as the fasting study as described above.

4. Importance of bioavailability and bioequivalence studies

4.1 Universal approach about comparative bioavailability

Most bioavailability studies, whether for a new or generic product, are carried out for the common theme. These studies are conducted to identify the quantitative nature of a specific product comparison. The absolute bioavailability of new drug is used to assess the pharmacokinetic parameters of an oral formulation relative to that of an intravenous dose or performance of a modified release formulation in comparison to a conventional capsule. For a generic product, it is mainly done for comparison of a competitive formulation with a reference or standard drug. Such commonality in comparative bioavailability studies suggests a universal experimental approach.

4.2 Comparative bioavailability studies of new drugs (NDA)

Comparative bioavailability studies for new drug are used to conduct to determine the bioavailability and bioequivalence of the formulation in humans for safety and efficacy. Information about bioavailability of new drug formulation is obtained by comparing the pharmacokinetics parameters of an intravenous and oral administration of new drug formulations having the same dose [26].

4.3 Comparative bioavailability of generic drugs (ANDA)

When a manufacturer wishes to gain therapeutic equivalence for introducing a competitive generic product into the market place, it is not necessary to conduct the full batch of clinical trials needed for the first product. If therapeutic equivalence has been determined, study has to be carried out according to prescribed study requirements, and it should be similar or equivalent to the previous or innovator product. This is regarded as therapeutically equivalent to the innovative drug product [27].

4.4 Testing under fasting conditions or fed conditions

When the particular drug is not showing any expected results under fasting conditions, then the drug can also be tested under fed conditions to meet all conditions as per regulatory norms in bioequivalence studies.

5. Conclusion

The concept of bioavailability and bioequivalence studies has been adopted by the pharmaceutical industry and national regulatory authorities throughout the world over 20 years. It is mainly due to increasing the number of generic drugs and its formulations and marketed after regulatory acceptance. So, the bioavailability and bioequivalence studies carried under stringent protocols and modified according to the needs. Pharmacokinetic parameters are evaluated by the statistical methods to get accurate results to assure high quality interchangeable and affordable drugs. There is a continuing attempts made by different organizations, authorities, and basic scientists to understand and develop more efficient and scientific valid approaches to evaluate bioavailability and bioequivalence studies of various formulations.

Author details

Divvela Hema Nagadurga
Avanthi Institute of Pharmaceutical Sciences, Visakhapatnam, India

*Address all correspondence to: mylabathulah@gmail.com

References

[1] Midhal KK, McKay G. Bioequivalence: Its history, practice, and future. AAPS Journal. 2009;**11**:664-670

[2] Boix-Montanes A. Relevance of equivalence assessment of topical products based on the pharmacokinetics approach. The European Journal of Pharmaceutical Sciences. 2011;**42**:173-179

[3] Skelly JP. A history of bio pharmaceutics in the food and drug administration. AAPS Journal. 2010;**12**:44-50

[4] Midha KK, Rawson MJ, Hubbard JW. The bioequivalence of highly variable drugs and drug products. The International Journal of Clinical Pharmacology and Therapeutics. 2005;**43**:485-498

[5] Chen ML, Lesko LJ. Individual bioequivalence revisited. Clinical Pharmacokinetics. 2001;**40**:701-706

[6] Lamy PP. Generic equivalents: Issues and concerns. The Journal of Clinical Pharmacology. 1986;**26**:309-316

[7] Food and Drug Administration (FDA). Guidance for industry: Statistical Procedures for Bioequivalence Studies Using a Standard Two-treatment Crossover Design. U.S Department of Health and Human Services. Food and Drug Administration, Center for Drug Evaluation and Research (CDER). July 1992. Available from: www.fda.gov/downloads/Drugs/Guidance ComplianceRegulatoryInformation/Guidance/ucm07244.pdf

[8] Food and Drug Administration (FDA). Guidance for Industry, Waiver of *In Vivo* Bioavailability and Bioequivalence Studies for Immediate-Release Solid Oral Dosage Forms Based on a Biopharmaceutics Classification System. U.S Department of Health and Human Services. Food and Drug Administration, Center for Drug Evaluation and Research (CDER). 2000. Available from: www.fda.gov/downloads/Drugs/GuidanceCompliance RegulatoryInformation/Guidance/ucm07246.pdf

[9] Food and Drug Administration (FDA). Guidance for Industry, Bio-analytical Method Validation. U.S Department of Health and Human Services. Food and Drug Administration, Center for Drug Evaluation and Research (CDER). Center for Veterinary Medicine (CVM). May 2001. Available from: www.fda.gov/downloads/Drugs/GuidanceCompliance RegulatoryInformation/Guidance/ucm070107.pdf

[10] Food and Drug Administration (FDA). Bioavailability and Bioequivalence Requirement. U.S Department of Health and Human Services. Food and Drug Administration, Center for Drug Evaluation and Research (CDER). Center for Veterinary Medicine (CVM). 2011. Available from: www.accessdata.fda.gov/scripts/cdrh/cfdocs/cfcf/cfsearch.cfem?Cfrpart=320

[11] Central Drugs Standard Control Organization (CDSCO). Guidelines for Bioavailability and Bioequivalence Studies. Directorate General of Health Service Ministry of Health and Family Welfare, Government of India, New Delhi. 2005. Available from: http://cdsco.nic.in/html/BE%20Guidelines%20Draft%over10%20march2005.pdf

[12] Chereson R. Bioavailability, bioequivalence, and drug selection. Basic Pharmacokinetics. 1997;**4**(8):1-21

[13] Ahmed AN, El Gamal S, Naggar V. Bioavailability: A pharmaceutical review. Journal of Novel Drug Delivery Technology. 2011:77-88

[14] Guidance for Industry Bioavailability and Bioequivalence Studies for Orally Administered Drug Products General Considerations. U.S Department of Health and Human Services. Food and Drug Administration, Center for Drug Evaluation and Research (CDER). 2001. Available from: http://www.fda.gov/downloads/Drugs/GuidanceComplianceRegulatoryInformation/Guidance/uc154838.pdf

[15] Pidgen A. Bioequivalence and generic prescribing: An industrial view. The Journal of Pharmacy and Pharmacology. 1996;**48**:11-16

[16] Food and Drug Administration (FDA). Guidance for Industry, Statistical Approaches to Establishing Bioequivalence. U.S Department of Health and Human Services. Food and Drug Administration, Center for Drug Evaluation and Research (CDER). 2001. Available from: www.fda.gov/downloads/Drugs/GuidanceComplianceRegulatoryInformation/Guidance/ucm07244.pdf

[17] Foood and Drug Administration (FDA). Guidance for Industry, Bioavailability and Bioequivalence Studies for Orally Administered Drug Products—General Considerations. U.S Department of Health and Human Services. Food and Drug Administration, Center for Drug Evaluation and Research (CDER). 2003. Available from: www.fda.gov/downloads/Drugs/GuidanceComplianceRegulatoryInformation/Guidance/ucm072878.pdf

[18] Bioequivalence Requirements Guidelines. Kingdom of Saudi Arabia: Saudi Food and Drug Authority Drug Sector. 2005. pp. 5-8. Available on: http://www.sfda.gov.sa

[19] Asian Guideline for the Conduct Bioavailability & Bioequivalence Studies. 2004. pp. 5-10

[20] Health Canada. Conduct and Analysis of Bioavailability and Bioequivalence Studies: Part A: Oral Dosage Formulations Used for Systemic Effects (1992); Part B: Oral Modified Release Formulations (1996); Report C: Report on Bioavailability of Oral Dosage Formulations, Not in Modified Release Form, or Drugs Used for Systemic Effects, Having Complicated or Variable Pharmacokinetics (1992). Health Products and Food Branch Guidence Document. 1992-1996. Available from: http://www.hc.sc.gc.ca

[21] Satoskar RS, Bhandarakar SD, Ainapure V. Pharmacology and pharmacotherapeutics. Popular Prakashan. 2001;**17**:10-11

[22] Löbenberg R, Amidon GL. Modern bioavailability, bioequivalence and biopharmaceutics classification system. New scientific approaches to international regulatory standards. European Journal of Pharmaceutics and Biopharmaceutics. 2000;**50**:3-12

[23] Qayyum A. Bioequivalence studies. National University of Sciences and Technology Pakistan. 2012;**39**:5-9

[24] Thiessen JJ. Bioavailability and bioequivalence. 2002;**57**:58

[25] Mastan S, Latha TB, Ajay S. The basic regulatory considerations and prospects for conducting bioavailability/bioequivalence (BA/BE) studies—An overview. Comparative Effectiveness Research. 2011;**1**:1-25

[26] Guideline for Bioequivalence Studies of Generic Products for Topical Use. 2003. pp. 6-10

[27] Chen M-L, Shah V, Patnaik R, Adams W, Hussain A, Conner D, et al. Bioavailability and bioequivalence: An FDA regulatory overview. Pharmaceutical Research. 2001;**18**(12):1645-1650

Section 3

Drug Delivery System

Chapter 5

pH-Responsive Microgels: Promising Carriers for Controlled Drug Delivery

Zermina Rashid

Abstract

The development of a new drug entity is a time-consuming and an expensive process; therefore, the design of new drug delivery systems for an existing drug molecule can significantly improve the safety and efficacy of the drug with improved patient compliance. In recent years, polymeric carriers have been widely investigated and are playing an important role in controlled drug delivery, biomedical applications, and tissue engineering. Microgels are microscopic hydrogels and have attracted much attention as vehicle for drug delivery. Stimuli-responsive MGs are smart drug delivery carriers and have the capability to incorporate and release their host molecules in response to stimuli (pH, ionic strength, and temperature), for targeted drug delivery. Of the many stimuli, alteration in pH is markedly fascinating because of the availability of pH gradients admissible for drug targeting. For example, pH gradients between normal tissues and some pathological sites between the extracellular environment and some cellular compartments, and along the gastrointestinal (GI) tract, are well characterized. Microgels can be fabricated through different methods.

Keywords: controlled drug delivery, microgels, stimuli-responsive microgels, targeted delivery, pharmaceutical applications, types, methods of formulation

1. Introduction

Among the available biomaterials, hydrogels, three-dimensional polymeric networks capable of imbibing large amounts of water or biological fluids, have proved their value in diverse biomedical applications [1–3]. In addition to the swelling property of the hydrogels, their biocompatibility, good mechanical properties, tunable chemical structure, and three-dimensional physical structure have made them one of the promising class of materials for tissue engineering [4, 5], pharmaceutical applications [6, 7], and biomaterials science [8]. In recent years, with the advancements in technology, interest in microscopic (microgels) and nanoscopic hydrogels (nanogels) has increased [9, 10].

Microgels, hydrogel particles formed by physical or chemical cross-linking of polymer networks in microscale size [11], have exceptional properties like large surface area, tunable size from micrometers to nanometers, ease in synthesis, control over particle size, responsiveness to environmental factors, and an interior network for the incorporation of therapeutic agents [12, 13].

 IntechOpen

2. Stimuli-responsive microgels

Stimuli-responsive properties can be incorporated into gels. Microgels may respond to a number of stimuli like pH, ionic strength, specific ions, external fields, and temperature [14–17]. Such DDSs are designed whether to target tissues, to reach specific intracellular locations, or to promote drug release [18]. Brief overview of the types of stimuli-responsive microgels is given below.

2.1 Types of stimuli-responsive microgels

2.1.1 Microgels responsive to temperature

Several classes of polymers, including poly(N-isopropylacrylamide) and poly(ethylene glycol), demonstrate swelling/deswelling changes in response to temperature [19, 20]. With increase in temperature, these systems have reduced solvency and pronounced deswelling. Nolan et al. [21] demonstrated higher insulin release from poly (N-isopropyl acrylamide), with increasing temperature. Temperature-dependent aggregation property of such thermosensitive microgel systems may also be utilized in drug delivery, e.g., at elevated temperature; due to aggregation of PNIPAM microgels particle inside the cancerous cell, toxicity was observed [22].

2.1.2 Microgels responsive to particular compounds

Microgels can be designed to be triggered by the concentration of particular compounds, like insulin [23, 24]. For example, insulin containing poly (diethyl aminoethyl methacrylate) microgels conjugated with glucose oxidase [25]. The enzymatic conversion of glucose to gluconic acid causes pH-responsive swelling of the polymer network leading to release of insulin. In another study Sui et al. [26] reported trifluoperazine triggered volume transition in calmodulin-based hydrogels.

2.1.3 Microgels responsive to external fields

Microgel systems may also respond to external fields (ultrasound, light, and magnetic fields). Patnaik et al. [27] investigated photoresponsive drug release in azo-dextran nanogels based on (trans-cis) photoisomerization of an azobenzene present in the cross-linker. For this system, the release of drug was slower for trans-configuration while faster for cis-configuration.

Metal nanoparticles may be used for optical or magnetic heating. When temperature-responsive microgels are combined with metals, heat induced by the external fields may result in deswelling, leading to release of the absorbed drugs. Using this perspective, Wong et al. [28] explored Fe-containing PNIPAM microgels. The microgels showed ability to manifest local heating attributed to an oscillating magnetic field. With increasing temperature microgels deswelled. Similar kind of triggering was also manifested in other studies, where light-originated heating of absorbed metal nanoparticles was used to induce local heat, provoking permeability variations in temperature-responsive polymers [29–31].

2.1.4 Microgels responsive to degradation

Microgel degradation in response to stimuli offers another way of controlled drug delivery [32, 33]. Such systems are commonly based on biodegradable microgels, occasionally surrounded by a shell impermeable to the drug. In later case, microgel degradation causes increased osmotic pressure, finally breaking the shell and drug release. Examples include dextran microgels coated by different polyelectrolyte multilayer systems [34] and lipid-coated microgels for the release of doxorubicin [35].

Biodegradable acrylamide/bisacrylamide microgels containing acetal linkers were investigated by Murthy et al. [36]. Biodegradation stimulated by low pH, resulting from acid-catalyzed hydrolysis of acetal linkage, was responsible for drug release. Similarly, Bromberg et al. [37] investigated poly (acrylic acid)-containing microgels cross-linked with disulfide groups. The chemical reduction of the disulfide bonds manifested the swelling of these systems.

2.1.5 Microgels responsive to pH

pH-responsive microgels represent one of the major approaches for microgel-based delivery of biomacromolecular drugs. Of the many stimuli, alteration in pH is markedly fascinating because of the availability of pH gradients admissible for drug targeting. For example, pH gradients between normal tissues and some pathological sites, between the extracellular environment and some cellular compartments, and along the gastrointestinal (GI) tract are well characterized [38]. Orally administered drug encounters a pH gradient as it move from the stomach (pH 1–2, fasted state) to the duodenum (pH of about 6) and along the jejunum and ileum (pH 6–7.5) [39, 40]; therefore, attempts to avoid deterioration of drug and/or to promote intestinal absorption by exploiting this pH gradient is promising. pH-responsive polymeric networks, hence, have been extensively studied for the design of efficient carriers for drug delivery [41].

pH-responsive polymers are generally fabricated by inserting pendant acidic or basic functional groups to the backbone of the polymer. These functional groups either accept or release protons in response to appropriate pH and changes in the ionic strength of the surrounding aqueous media [42]. Polymers with acidic groups are unexpanded at low pH values, since the acidic groups are protonated and unionized. While increasing pH acidic groups are ionized, the resulting negatively charged polymer expands. The opposite behavior will be observed in the case of polybasic polymers [43, 44]. These systems can form polyelectrolytes with water, and microgels fabricated from weak polyelectrolytes demonstrate a pH-responsive volume phase changes. On the basis of the framework of polyelectrolyte, pH-responsive microgels can be classified as cationic, basic, or amphoteric. For instance, poly(acrylic acid) and polyethylenimine are weak polyacid and a polybase, respectively.

3. Synthesis of microgels

Methods used for the synthesis of microgels can be divided into two major ideas:

(a) The synthesis of microgels in homogeneous phase

(b) The synthesis of microgels in heterophase

3.1 Synthesis of microgels in homogeneous phase

The first approach is based on the investigations of Staudinger [45], who prepared inter- and intramolecularly cross-linked microgels by free radical cross-linking copolymerization of monomers in dilute solutions. However, the resulting internal structure of microgels was not well established, but investigations performed on these systems were key step to understand the process of gel formation [46].

Other techniques include coacervation and desolvation. In both techniques phase separation of readily formed polymers takes place, resulting in micro-/nanoparticles which are then cross-linked. **Figure 1** represents typical steps involved in coacervation method. Phase separation is usually induced by changing temperature, adding salt, nonsolvent addition, non-compatible polymer addition, or polymer-polymer interaction. The resulting coacervate (polymer droplet) is then solidified and stabilized forming microgel particle. This technique is usually employed in synthesis of microgels from biopolymers such as (modified) gelatin or chitosan. For example, pH-responsive chitosan nanoparticles were synthesized by complex coacervation [47] and two-step desolvation route was involved in synthesis of gelatin nanoparticles [48].

3.2 Synthesis of microgel in heterogeneous phase

Heterophase copolymerization of monomers with cross-linking agents in aqueous solution can be distinguished as:

- Dispersion/precipitation polymerization
- Miniemulsion polymerization
- Microemulsion polymerization

3.2.1 Dispersion/precipitation polymerization

In this technique, polymerization generally starts in a homogenous solution of monomers and cross-linkers [49, 50]; as polymerization progresses, the monomer and the developed oligomers remain soluble; after achieving the critical length phase, separation takes place by enthalpic precipitation leading to particle nuclei formation. The nuclei aggregate to form large particles that carry on growing resulting into microgel formation. In dispersion polymerization stabilizers can be added to regulate the particle size and to keep particles in narrow size distribution [51]. The described method is schematically presented in **Figure 2**.

Dispersion polymerization technique was employed for the synthesis of pH-sensitive poly((2-dimethylamino)ethyl methacrylate) microgels with diameter of about 100–200 nm in dry sate [52]. The microgels exhibited volume phase change at about pH 8, with 32 times decrease in diameter. Dispersion polymerization was involved in the preparation of hydrophilic microparticles of poly(2-hydroxyethyl methacrylate) [53].

Duracher et al. [54] synthesized thermoresponsive microgels by precipitation polymerization of N-isopropylmethacrylamide. The prepared microgels were

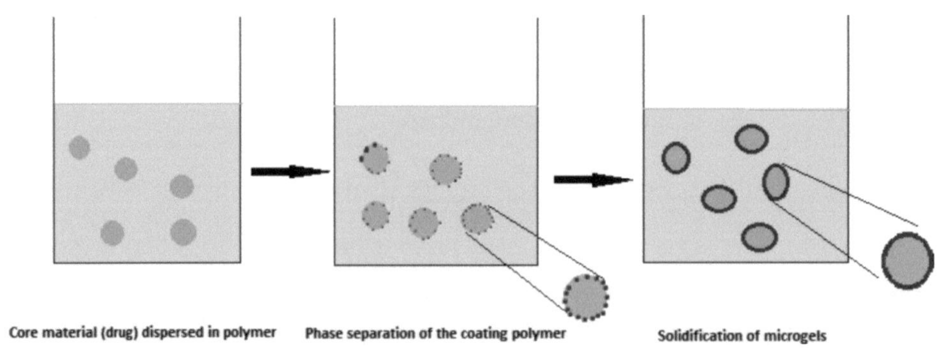

Figure 1.
Schematic presentation of coacervation technique.

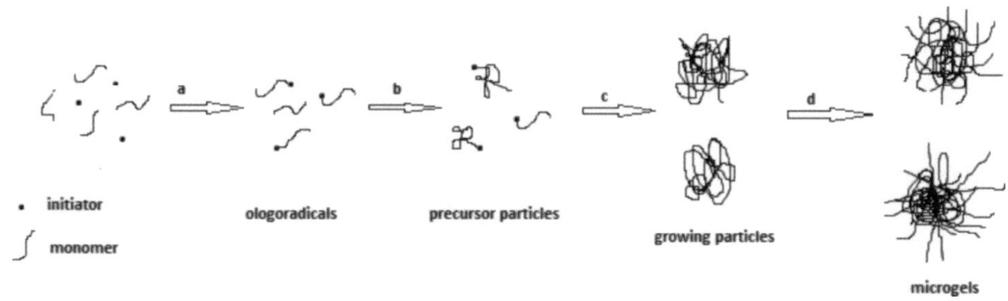

Figure 2.
Precipitation polymerization (a) initiation of polymerization and chain growth, (b) precipitation and nuclei formation, (c) particle growth, and (d) microgels.

found to be temperature sensitive. Moreover, with the modifications in the synthetic protocol, more complex microgel structures can be synthesized. Examples include temperature- and pH-sensitive microgels prepared by copolymerization of N-isopropylmethacrylamide with acrylic acid [55], vinyl acetic acid [56, 57], or 2-aminoethyl methacrylate hydrochloride [58].

One approach to synthesize complex structures, e.g., core-shell microgels or hollow microgels, involves polymerization of different monomers and/or already formed seed particle. Core-shell microgels have structurally separated zones of different polymers. Zhou et al. [59] synthesized temperature sensitive microgels based on oligo(ethylene glycol). The microgels were stable across the important physiological temperature range with adjustable volume phase changes.

3.2.2 Synthesis of microgels in microemulsions

In general, microemulsions can be prepared as direct oil-in-water (O/W) or inverse water-in-oil (W/O) emulsions. The inverse emulsions are widely investigated for the formulation of hydrogel nanoparticles. In this approach, dispersed phase consists of either monomer having ability to polymerize or prepolymers with ability of cross-linking dissolved in water is added to a continuous phase of organic medium having large amount of oil-soluble surfactant. The mixture is stirred to achieve thermodynamically stable microemulsion. Synthesis of microgels takes place inside the droplets, e.g., via free radical polymerization. Initiation of polymerization takes place either from the interior of droplets or from the continuous phase [60]. **Figure 3** illustrates the microgel synthesis in W/O emulsion.

Shen et al. [61] synthesized poly(acrylamide-co-acrylic acid) microgels by polymerization in inverse microemulsion. The effect of chemical constitution on size, morphology, swelling behavior, thermal properties, and pH-sensitivity was explored. The size of p(AM-co-AA) microgels was larger in comparison to PAM microgels. The microgels exhibited pH-responsive behavior and have higher swelling ratio, with an increase in acrylic acid content.

In another study, microemulsion polymerization phenomenon was employed for the copolymerization of methacrylic acid and 2-ethylhexyl acrylate to demonstrate colon-specific delivery of drug. An anticancer drug (5-fluorouracil) was entrapped inside the copolymer through solvent evaporation method. In vitro drug release studies performed at different pH levels revealed pH-dependent release of 5-fluorouracil in a sustained manner [62].

3.2.3 Microgel synthesis in miniemulsions

Miniemulsions in general are kinetically stable emulsions; considerably less surfactant is required for the droplet stabilization [63]. This approach is versatile

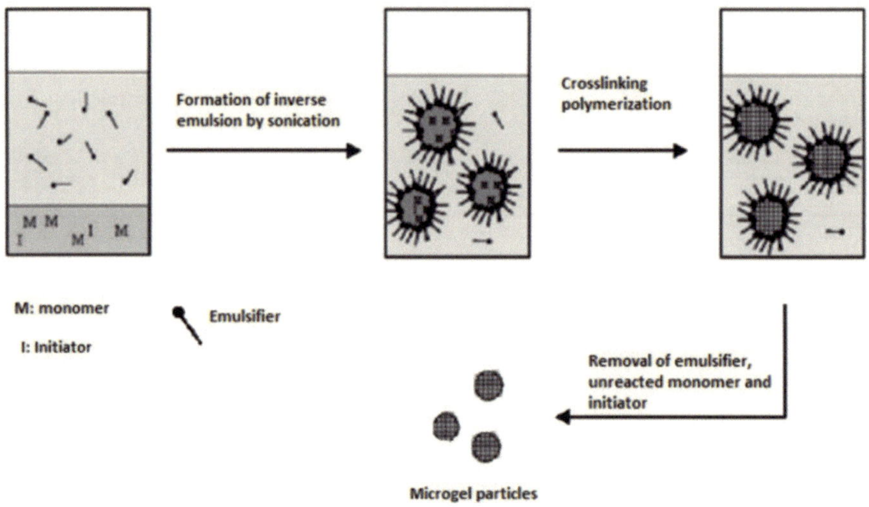

Figure 3.
Illustration of microgel preparation via inverse emulsion polymerization.

and allows utilization of different monomers, functional compounds incorporation, and the accurate adaptation of droplets and particles size [64, 65]. In general, high deformation forces are applied to pre-emulsion of droplet leading to uniform distribution of well-defined nanodroplets (50–500 nm). The surfactant present in the system obstructs the coalescence of these nanodroplets; in addition, the costablizer added to dispersed phase prevents Ostwald ripening leading to kinetically stable miniemulsion [66].

Miniemulsions can be classified as direct (oil-in-water) or inverse (water-in-oil) systems. Oil-in-water miniemulsification is a well-established approach for the polymerization of hydrophobic monomers for the formulation of polymeric latexes [63]; on the other hand, the inverse method involves diverse synthetic pathways for the formation of nanohydrogels [67]. One approach involves the free radical copolymerization of hydrophilic monomers with cross-linking agents in dispersed droplets

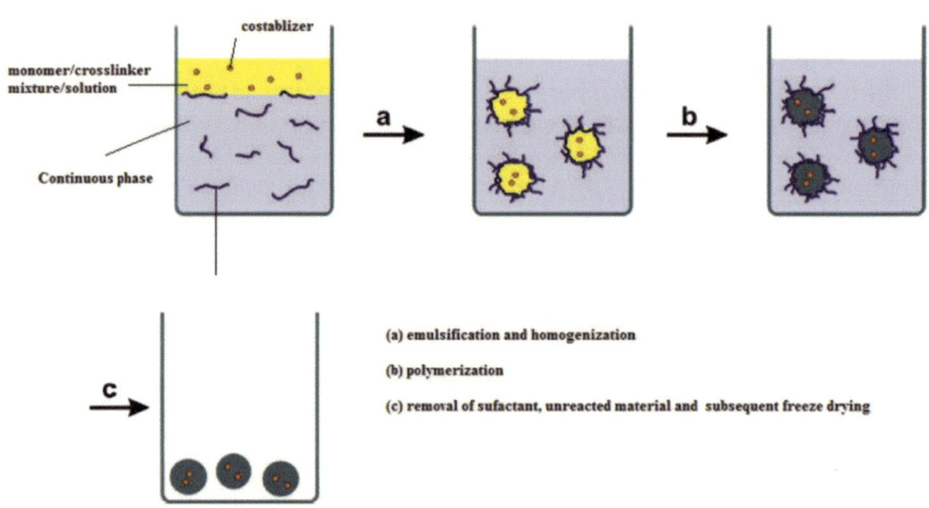

Figure 4.
Schematic illustration of radical cross-linking in inverse miniemulsion.

of either aqueous solutions of these compounds or their mixture without additional solvent. The monomers must be immiscible with the continuous phase. Examples include the formation of polyacrylamide (PAAm)- [68] and PHEMA-based [65] microgels. **Figure 4** schematically represents the described synthetic pathway.

Another approach is cross-linking of preformed polymers in inverse miniemulsion. In this method mixture of two W/O emulsions (A and B) are ultrasonicated. Emulsion A constitutes the solution of already formed polymer, and emulsion B constitutes solution of cross-linker. Ultrasonication leads to mixing of the components of both emulsions, inducing the cross-linking reaction. This method has been employed for the synthesis of covalently cross-linked gelatin microgels [69]. In another study, temperature-responsive nanogels poly(N-isopropylacrylamide) nanogels were fabricated by nanoemulsion polymerization as smart delivery systems [70].

4. Pharmaceutical applications of pH-responsive microgels

pH-responsive microgels have demonstrated a number of medical applications (**Table 1**). Few examples from the literature are demonstrated here.

pH-responsive p(NIPAAm/AA) microgels were fabricated for transferrin-based targeting of cancer [71]. These microgels were able for specific delivery to human cervical carcinoma cell line (HeLa) cells. In another study methacrylic-based copolymeric pH-sensitive nanogels were prepared for targeted delivery of 5-fluorouracil to the colon [62]. Recently, Eswaramma et al. [72] developed pH-sensitive interpenetrating polymer network (IPN) microgels of chitosan and guar gum-*g*-poly((2-dimethylamino)ethyl methacrylate) (GG-*g*-PDMAEMA) and treated as responsive drug carriers for an anticancer agent, 5-fluorouracil (5-FU). The microgels showed encapsulation efficiency up to 81%, and the release kinetics showed pH-dependent drug release with an excellent controlled release pattern for 5-FU over a period of more than 24 h.

Dadsetan et al. [73] used a copolymer of oligo(poly(ethylene glycol) fumarate) (OPF) and sodium methacrylate (SMA) to fabricate the pH-responsive microgels for the delivery of doxorubicin (DOX) in order to optimize its antitumor activity

Polymers	Polymeric DDSs	Drug	Application	Reference
GG-*g*-PDMAEMA	IPN-Microgels	5 fluorouracil	Antitumor activity	[72]
OPF-SMA microgels	Microgels	Doxorubicin	Antitumor activity	[73]
MEMA-co-IA	Microgels	Esomeprazole	Intestinal delivery	[76]
P(MMA-*g*-EG)	Microgels	Insulin	Oral peptide delivery	[82]
P(AM)-g-carrageenan and sodium alginate	Hydrogel beads	Ketoprofen	For colon-targeted delivery	[83]
Methacrylate derivatives of dextran and concanavalin	Microgels	Insulin	Self-regulated insulin delivery	[84]
Alg and chemically modified carboxymethyl CS	Microgels	Protein drug	For oral delivery	[85]

Table 1.
Examples of various applications of microgels as drug delivery carriers.

while minimizing its systemic toxicity. The resulting microgels exhibited sensitivity to the pH and ionic strength of the surrounding environment and demonstrated that DOX was efficiently loaded into the microgels and released in a controlled fashion via an ion exchange mechanism. The antitumor activity of the released DOX was assessed using a human chordoma cell line revealed that OPF-SMA microgels prolonged the cell-killing effect of DOX.

Tripahi et al. [74] developed a pH-sensitive intragastric floating polymer microgel beads containing clarithromycin for the treatment of peptic ulcer. The optimized formulation successfully maintained minimum inhibition concentration of clarithromycin at the infection site and potentially allowed penetration of the drug inside the mucus gel. Varma et al. [75] have chemically modified guar gum (GG) as a pH-sensitive copolymer and formulated intestinal-targeting esomeprazole magnesium (ESO) nanoparticles (NPs). Polyacrylamide-grafted guar gum copolymer was synthesized by free radical polymerization, and ESO-loaded pH-sensitive NPs were prepared by nanoemulsification polymer cross-linking method. In vitro release studies showed pH-dependent drug release. The pH-sensitive NPs resisted drug release in acidic pH and delayed the release in alkaline environment.

In another study novel pH-responsive poly(methoxyethyl metacrylate-co-itaconic acid) microgels were fabricated and evaluated for controlled and extended delivery of model acid labile drug (esomeprazole). The designed microgels successfully protected the drug from acidic environment of the stomach, with potential intestinal drug delivery over an extended period of time. Thus, suggesting p(MEMA-co-IA) micro-hydrogels as good candidate of an orally administrated site-specific and controlled drug delivery system, such as proton-pump inhibitors, proteins, and peptides [76]. In similar studies p(hydroxyethyl methacrylate-co-itaconic acid) microgels, poly(2-ethyl hexyl acrylate-co-IA) microgels, and poly(butyl acrylate-co-itaconic acid) microgels showed pH-responsive swelling and drug release behavior with maximum release at pH 7.4 and negligible release at pH 1.2 suggesting the potential use of these drug delivery system for oral intestinal delivery of therapeutics [77–79].

A novel 5-aminosalicylic acid (5-ASA)-loaded pH-sensitive poly(methoxy ethylene glycol-caprolactone-co-methacrylic acid-co-poly(ethylene glycol) dimethacrylate) microgels were prepared for treatment of ulcerative colitis. The microgels were found to be shrunk at pH 1.2 and expanded at pH 7.4. Safety evaluation of microgels was conducted by maximum tolerated dose (MTD) method. The 5-ASA/microgels were used to treat ulcerative colitis in mice, and free 5-ASA was used as positive control. It was found that 5-ASA has good efficacy for treating ulcerative colitis, and microgels entrapping 5-ASA could significantly enhance the colon targeting to improve its efficacy [80].

Xua et al. [81] fabricated novel biodegradable and pH-sensitive microgels based on poly(ε-caprolactone)-pluronic-poly(ε-caprolactone)-dimethacrylate, methyl acrylic acid, and poly(ethylene glycol)dimethacrylate cross-linked with N,N′-methylenebisacrylamide. Hydrophilic model drug (vitamin B12) was loaded to investigate in vitro release profile; the developed drug delivery system demonstrated pH-sensitive drug release behavior.

Lowman et al. [82] studied the use of poly(methacrylic-*g*-ethylene glycol) (P(MMA-*g*-EG)), a hydrogel microparticle that responds to a change in pH for the transport of orally administered insulin. This drug is a peptide labile to proteolytic degradation in the acidic stomach. Thus this pH-responsive carrier protected insulin in the acidic environment of the stomach as a result of the intermolecular interaction that prevented the hydrogel from swelling. But once the microparticles reached alkaline and neutral environments, namely, the intestine, the interaction that occurred previously was lost, and the pore size of the hydrogel increased, thus allowing insulin release.

5. Conclusion

This chapter has attempted the compilation of the advances in the field of stimuli-responsive microgel technology and their application in controlled release drug delivery carriers. The ultimate goal for controlled drug release is to maximize therapeutic activity while minimizing the negative side effects of the drug. In this regard, versatile micro- and nanoscale delivery approaches based on smart polymers have already been established to seek the distinct advantages in drug delivery. However, the new polymers and nanocarriers definitely require extensive consideration of toxicological and immunological issues, which are often ignored during the research phase.

Conflict of interest

There is no conflict of interest.

Author details

Zermina Rashid
Department of Pharmacy, The Women University, Multan, Pakistan

*Address all correspondence to: zermina_malik@yahoo.com

References

[1] Philip AK, Philip B. Colon targeted drug delivery systems: A review on primary and novel approaches. Oman Medical Journal. 2010;**25**:79-97

[2] Peppas NA, Huang Y, Torres-Lugo M, Ward JH, Zhange J. Physiochemical foundation and structure design of hydrogel in medicine and biology. Annual Review of Biomedical Engineering. 2000;**2**:9-29

[3] Hoffman AS. Hydrogels for biomedical applications. Advanced Drug Delivery Reviews. 2002;**54**:3-12

[4] Drury JL, Mooney DJ. Hydrogels for tissue engineering: Scaffold design variables and applications. Biomaterials. 2003;**24**:4337-4351

[5] Nguyen KT, West JL. Photo-polymerizable hydrogels for tissue engineering applications. Biomaterials. 2002;**23**:4307-4314

[6] Yeomans K. Hydrogels-very versatile materials. Chemical Reviews. 2000;**10**:2-5

[7] Kim SW, Bae Y, Okano T. Hydrogels: Swelling, drug loading, and release. Pharmaceutical Research. 1992;**9**:283-290

[8] Kim JJ, Park K. Smart hydrogels for bioseparation. Bioseparation. 1998;7:177-184

[9] Kingsley JD, Dou H, Morehead J, Rainbow B, Gendelman HE, Destache CJ. Nanotechnology: A focus on nanoparticles as a drug delivery system. Journal of Neuroimmune Pharmacology. 2006;**1**:340-350

[10] Nahar M, Dutta T, Murugesan S, Asthana A, Mishra D, Rajkumar V, et al. Functional polymeric nanoparticles: An efficient and promising tool for active delivery of bioactives. Critical Reviews in Therapeutic Drug Carrier Systems. 2006;**23**:259-318

[11] Vinogradov SV, Kabanov AV. Nanogels as pharmaceutical carriers: Finite networks of infinite capabilities. Angewandte Chemie, International Edition. 2009;**48**:5418-5429

[12] Oh JK, Drumright R, Siegwart DJ, Matyjaszewski K. The development of microgels/nanogels for drug delivery applications. Progress in Polymer Sciences. 2008;**33**:448-477

[13] Soussan E, Cassel S, Blanzat M, Rico-Lattes I. Drug delivery by soft matter: Matrix and vesicular carriers. Angewandte Chemie International Edition in English. 2009;**48**:274-288

[14] Malmsten M, Bysell H, Hansson P. Biomacromolecules in microgels-opportunities and challenges for drug delivery. Current Opinion in Colloid and Interface Science. 2010;**15**:435-444

[15] Hendrickson GR, Smith MH, South AB, Lyon LA. Design of multiresponsive hydrogel particles and assemblies. Advanced Functional Materials. 2010;**20**:1697-1712

[16] Welsch N, Wittemann AW, Ballauff M. Enhanced activity of enzymes immobilized in thermoresponsive core-shell microgels. The Journal of Physical Chemistry. B. 2009;**113**:16039-16045

[17] Klinger D, Landfester K. Stimuli-responsive microgels for the loading and release of functional compounds: Fundamental concepts and applications. Polymer. 2012;**53**:5209-5231

[18] Stuart MAC, Huck WTS, Genzer J, Muller M, Ober C, Stamm M, et al. Emerging applications of stimuli-responsive polymer materials. Nature Materials. 2010;**9**:101-103

[19] Das M, Zhang H, Kumacheva E. Microgels: Old materials with new applications. Annual Review of Materials Research. 2006;**36**:117-142

[20] Napier ME, Desimone JM. Nanoparticle drug delivery platform. Polymer Reviews. 2007;**47**:321-327

[21] Nolan CM, Gelbaum LT, Lyon LA. 1H NMR investigation of thermally triggered insulin release from poly(N-isopropylacrylamide) microgels. Biomacromolecules. 2006;7:2918-2922

[22] Nayak S, Lee H, Chielewski J, Lyon LA. Folate-mediated cell targeting and cytotoxicity using thermoresponsive microgels. Journal of the American Chemical Society. 2004;**126**:10258-10259

[23] Miyata T, Jikihara A, Nakamae K, Hoffmann AS. Preparation of reversibly glucose-responsive hydrogels by covalent immobilization of lectin in polymer networks having pendant glucose. Journal of Biomaterials Science. Polymer Edition. 2004;**15**:1085-1098

[24] Kim JJ, Park K. Modulated insulin delivery from glucose-sensitive hydrogel dosage forms. Journal of Controlled Release. 2001;77:39-47

[25] Ito Y, Casolaro M, Kono K, Yukio I. An insulin-releasing system that is responsive to glucose. Journal of Controlled Release. 1989;**10**:195-203

[26] Sui Z, King WJ, Murphy WL. Dynamic materials based on a protein conformational change. Advanced Materials. 2007;**19**:3377-3380

[27] Patnaik S, Sharma AK, Garg BS, Gandhi RP, Gupta KC. Photoregulation of drug release in azo-dextran nanogels. International Journal of Pharmaceutics. 2007;**342**:184-193

[28] Wong JE, Gaharwar AK, Müller-Schulte D, Bahadur D, Richtering W. Dual-stimuli responsive PNiPAM microgel achieved via layer-by-layer assembly: Magnetic and thermoresponsive. Journal of Colloid and Interface Science. 2008;**324**:47-54

[29] Skirtach AG, Dejugnat C, Braun D, Susha AS, Rogach AL, Parak WJ, et al. The role of metal nanoparticles in remote release of encapsulated materials. Nano Letters. 2005;**5**:1371-1377

[30] Radt B, Smith TA, Caruso F. Optically addressable nanostructures capsules. Advanced Materials. 2004;**16**:2184-2189

[31] Angelatos AS, Radt B, Caruso F. Light-responsive polyelectrolyte/gold nanoparticle microcapsules. The Journal of Physical Chemistry. B. 2005;**109**:3071-3076

[32] Oh JK, Sieqwart DJ, Matyjaszewski K. Synthesis and biodegradation of nanogels as delivery carriers for carbohydrate drugs. Biomacromolecules. 2007;**8**:3326-3331

[33] Liu YY, Fan X-D, Kang T, Sun L. A cyclodextrin microgel for controlled release driven by inclusion effects. Macromolecular Rapid Communications. 2004;**25**:1912-1916

[34] Geest BGD, Dejugnat C, Prevot M, Sukhorukov GB, Demesteer J, De Smedt SC. Self-rupturing and hollow microcapsules prepared from biopolyelectrolyte-coated microgels. Advanced Functional Materials. 2007;**17**:531-537

[35] Kiser PF, Wilison G, Needham D. Lipid-coated microgels for the triggered release of doxorubicin. Journal of Controlled Release. 2000;**68**:9-22

[36] Murthy N, Xu M, Schuck S, Kunisawa J, Shastri N, Frechet JMJ. A macromolecular delivery vehicle for protein-based vaccines: Acid-degradable

protein loaded microgels. Proceedings of the National Academy of Sciences. 2003;**100**:4995-5000

[37] Bromberg L, Temchenko M, Alakhov V, Hatton TA. Kinetics of swelling of polyether-modified poly(acrylic acid) microgels with permanent and degradable cross-links. Langmuir. 2005;**21**:1590-1598

[38] Arnaud EF, Dufresne MH, Leroux JC. pH-sensitive vesicles, polymeric micelles, and nanospheres prepared with polycarboxylates. Advanced Drug Delivery Reviews. 2012;**64**:979-992

[39] Daugherty AL, Mrsny RJ. Transcellular uptake mechanisms of the intestinal epithelial barrier part one. Pharmaceutical Science and Technology Today. 1999;**4**:144-151

[40] Fallingborg J. Intraluminal pH of the human gastrointestinal tract. Danish Medical Bulletin. 1999;**46**:183-196

[41] Mahdi K, Masoud E, Parham SZ, Fereshteh M, Negar F, Zahra S, et al. pH-sensitive stimulus-responsive nanocarriers for targeted delivery of therapeutic agents. WIREs Nanomedicine and Nanobiotechnology. 2016;**8**:696-716. DOI: 10.1002/wnan.1389

[42] Langer R, Peppas NA. Advances in biomaterials, drug delivery and bionanotechnology. AICHE Journal. 2003;**49**:2990-3006

[43] Eichenbaum GM, Kiser PF, Dobrynin AV, Simon SA, Needham D. Investigation of the swelling response and loading of ionic microgels with drugs and proteins: The dependence on cross-link density. Macromolecules. 1999;**32**:4876-4878

[44] Yoshida T, Lai TC, Kwon GS, Sako K. pH- and ion-sensitive polymers for drug delivery. Expert Opinion on Drug Delivery. 2013;**10**:1497-1513

[45] Staudinger H, Husemann E. Berichte Der Deutschen Chemischen Gesellschaft. 1935;**68**:1618-1634

[46] Funke W, Okay O, Joos-Muller B. Microgels-intramolecularly crosslinked macromolecules with a globular structure. Advances in Polymer Science. 1998;**136**:139-234

[47] Zhou XLB, Yu X, Zha X, Zhang X, Chen Y, Wang X, et al. Controlled release of PEI/DNA complexes from mannose-bearing chitosan microspheres as a potent delivery system to enhance immune response to HBV DNA vaccine. Journal of Controlled Release. 2007;**121**:200-207

[48] Balthasar S, Michaelis K, Dinauer N, von Briesen H, Kreuter J, Langer K. Preparation and characterisation of antibody modified gelatin nanoparticles as drug carrier system for uptake in lymphocytes. Biomaterials. 2005;**26**:2723-2732

[49] Downey JS, Frank RS, Li WH, Stover HDH. Growth mechanism of poly(divinylbenzene) microsphere in precipitation polymerization. Macromolecules. 1999;**32**:2838-2844

[50] Kai L, Stover HDH. Synthesis of monodisperse poly(divinylbenzene) microsphere journal of polymer science part A-polymer. Chemistry. 1993;**31**:2473-2479

[51] Fitch RM. Non-aqueous dispersion. Journal of Elastomers and Plastics. 1971;**3**:146-156

[52] Emileh A, Vasheghani-Farahani E, Imani M. Preparation and characterization of pH-sensitive microgels of poly((2-dimethylamino) ethyl methacrylate). Macromolecular Symposia. 2007;**255**:1-7

[53] Ma Z, Lacroix-Desmazes P. Dispersion polymerization of 2-hydroxyethyl methacrylate

stabilized by a hydrophilic/CO_2-philic poly(ethylene oxide)-b-poly(1,1,2,2-tetrahydroperfluorodecyl acrylate) (PEO-b-PFDA) diblock copolymer in supercritical carbon dioxide. Polymer. 2004;**45**:6789-6797

[54] Duracher D, Elaïssari A, Pichot C. Preparation of poly(N-isopropylmethacrylamide) latexes kinetic studies and characterization. Journal of Polymer Science Part A: Polymer Chemistry. 1999;**37**:1823-1837

[55] Debord JD, Lyon LA. Synthesis and characterization of pH-responsive copolymer microgels with tunable volume phase transition temperatures. Langmuir. 2003;**19**:7662-7664

[56] Hofl S, Zitzler L, Hellweg T, Herminghaus S, Mugele F. Volume phase transition of "smart" microgels in bulk solution and adsorbed at an Interface: A combined AFM, dynamic light, and small angle neutron scattering study. Polymer. 2007;**48**:245-254

[57] Hoare T, Pelton R. Highly pH and temperature responsive microgels functionalized with vinylacetic acid. Macromolecules. 2004;**37**:2544-2550

[58] Lopez-Leon T, Ortega-Vinuesa JL, Bastos-Gonzalez D, Elaissari A. Cationic and anionic poly(N-isopropylacrylamide) based submicron gel particles: Electrokinetic properties and colloidal stability. The Journal of Physical Chemistry. B. 2006;**110**:4629-4636

[59] Zhou T, Weitai W, Shuiqin Z. Engineering oligo(ethylene glycol)-based thermosensitive microgels for drug delivery application. Polymer. 2010;**51**:3926-3933

[60] Corpart JM, Candau F. Formulation and polymerization of microemulsions containing a mixture of cationic and anionic monomers. Colloid and Polymer Science. 1993;**271**:1055-1067

[61] Shen Y, Zhang X, Jianjun L, Zhang A, Chen K, Xiaoqin L. Effect of chemical composition on properties of pH-responsive poly(acrylamide-co-acrylic acid) microgels prepared by inverse microemulsion polymerization. Colloids and Surfaces A: Physicochemical and Engineering Aspects. 2009;**350**:87-90

[62] Ashwanikumar N, Kumar NK, Nair SA, Kumar GV. Methacrylic-based nanogels for the pH-sensitive delivery of 5-fluorouracil in the colon. International Journal of Nanomedicine. 2012;**7**:5769-5779

[63] Landfester K. The generation of nanoparticles in miniemulsions. Advanced Materials. 2001;**13**:765-768

[64] Urban M, Musyanovych A, Landfester K. Fluorescent superparamagnetic polylactide nanoparticles by combination of miniemulsion and emulsion/solvent evaporation techniques. Macromolecular Chemistry and Physics. 2009;**210**:961-970

[65] Landfester K. Synthesis of colloidal particles in miniemulsions. Annual Review of Materials Research. 2006;**36**:231-279

[66] Landfester K, Willert M, Antonietti M. Preparation of polymer particles in nonaqueous direct and inverse miniemulsions. Macromolecules. 2000;**33**:2370-2376

[67] Tomalia DA. Birth of a new macromolecular architecture: Dendrimers as quantized building blocks for nanoscale synthetic polymer chemistry. Progress in Polymer Science. 2005;**30**:294-324

[68] Kobitskaya E, Ekinci D, Manzke A, Plettl A, Wiedwald U, Ziemann P. Narrowly size distributed zinc-containing poly(acrylamide) latexes via inverse miniemulsion polymerization. Macromolecules. 2010;**43**:3294-3305

[69] Ethirajan A, Schoeller K, Musyanovych A, Ziener U, Landfester K. Synthesis and optimization of gelatin nanoparticles using the miniemulsion process. Biomacromolecules. 2008;**9**:2383-2389

[70] TFuciños C, Fucinos P, Míguez M, Katime I, Pastrana LM, Rúa ML. Temperature- and pH-sensitive nanohydrogels of poly(N-isopropylacrylamide) for food packaging applications: Modelling the swelling-collapse behaviour. PLoS ONE. 2014;**9**:e87190. DOI: 10.1371

[71] Das M, Mardyani S, Chan WCW, Kumacheva E. Biofunctionalized pH responsive microgels for cancer cell targeting: Rational design. Advanced Materials. 2006;**18**:80-83

[72] Eswaramma S, Sivagangi Reddy N, Krishna Rao KSV. Carbohydrate polymer based pH-sensitive IPN microgels: Synthesis, characterization and drug release characteristics. Materials Chemistry and Physics. 2017;**195**:176-118

[73] Dadsetan M, Taylor KE, Yong C, Bajzer Z, Lu L, Yaszemski MJ. Controlled release of doxorubicin from pH-responsive microgels. Acta Biomaterialia. 2013;**9**(3):5438-5446

[74] Tripahi GK, Singh S, Nath G. Formulation and evaluation of pH sensitive polymeric blended microgel beads of clarithromycin for the effective treatment of helicobacter pylori. Der Pharmacia Sinica. 2010;**1**:245-255

[75] Varma VNSK, Shivakumar HG, Balamuralidhara V, Navya M, Hani U. Development of pH sensitive nanoparticles for intestinal drug delivery using chemically modified guar gum Co-polymer. Iranian Journal of Pharmaceutical Research. 2016;**15**:83-94

[76] Rashid Z, Ranjha NM, Razzaq R, Raza H. Fabrication and in vitro evaluation of novel pH-sensitive poly(2-methoxyethyl methacrylate-co-itaconic acid) microgels. Advances in Polymer Technology. 2018;**37**:1268-1277

[77] Rashid Z, Ranjha NM, Razzaq R, Raza H, Mehmood A. Preparation and evaluation of pH responsive poly (2-Hydroxyethyl methacrylate-co-Itaconic acid) microgels for controlled drug delivery. Acta Poloniae Pharmaceutica. 2016;**73**(4):1045-1055

[78] Razzaq R, Ranjha NM, Rashid Z, Raza H. Preparation and characterization of chemically crosslinked pH sensitive poly (2-ethyl hexyl acrylate-co- itaconic acid) microgels for controlled drug delivery of Diltiazem hydrochloride. Latin American Journal of Pharmacy. 2016;**35**(8):1754-1762

[79] Razzaq R, Ranjha NM, Rashid Z, Nasir B. Preparation and evaluation of novel pH-sensitive poly(butyl acrylate-*co*-itaconic acid) hydrogel microspheres for controlled drug delivery. Advances in Polymer Technology. 2018;**37**(1) 21663(1-9)

[80] Xu X, Gu YC, Tang XH, Qian ZY. Preparation of 5-Aminosalicylic acid-loaded pH-sensitive P(CE-MAA-EG) microgels for the treatment of ulcerative colitis. Science of Advanced Materials. 2013;**5**:86-86

[81] Xua X, Fu S, Wang K, Jia W, Guo G, Zheng X, et al. Preparation and characterization of Vitamin-12 loaded biodegradable pH-sensitive microgels. Journal of Microencapsulation. Micro and Nano Carriers. 2009;**26**:642-648

[82] Lowman AM, Morishita M, Kajita M, Nagai T, Peppas NJ. Oral delivery of insulin using pH-responsive complexation gels. Journal of Pharmaceutical Sciences. 1999;**88**:933-937

[83] Kulkarni RV, Boppana R, Krishna MG, Mutalik S, Kaiyane VK. pH responsive interpenetrating network hydrogel beads of poly(acrylamide)-g-carrageenan and sodium alginate for intestinal targeted drug delivery: Synthesis, in vitro and in vivo evaluation. Journal of Colloid and Interface Science. 2012;**367**:509-517

[84] Yin R, Tong Z, Yang D, Nie J. Glucose and pH dual-responsive concanavalin a based microhydrogels for insulin delivery. International Journal of Biological Macromolecules. 2011;**49**:1137-1142

[85] El-Sherbiny IM. Enhanced pH-responsive carrier system based on alginate and chemically modified carboxymethyl chitosan for oral delivery of protein drugs: Preparation and *in-vitro* assessment. Carbohydrate Polymers. 2010;**80**:1125-1136

Chapter 6

Using Microbubbles as Targeted Drug Delivery to Improve AIDS

Harsha Virsingh Sonaye, Rafik Yakub Shaikh and Chandrashekhar A. Doifode

Abstract

No preventive vaccines are available for the treatment of AIDS. To improve therapy, combinational antiretroviral drugs are given; however some patients develop resistance to particular combinational drug. Microbubble-mediated drug delivery technology solves the problem by reducing systemic dose and toxicity. Microbubbles are bubbles smaller than one millimeter in diameter but larger than one micrometer. The general composition of microbubble is gas core. The mechanism of microbubbles through which its delivery increases is sonoporation, the formation of openings in the vasculature, induced by ultrasound-triggered oscillations and destruction of microbubbles. Rapid isolation strategy of CD4+ cells is mixing blood and glass microbubbles which then bind with the specific target cells to the microbubble carrying specific antibodies on their surface. The target cells will spontaneously float to the top of the blood vial and can be quickly separated. The microbubbles are particularly used in the diagnosis of AIDS because of their cell isolation techniques which is rapid and inexpensive and their small size to pass through capillary for perfusion in tissue This review demonstrates the problems with the current treatment of the disease and shed light on the remarkable potential of microbubbles to provide more effective treatment and prevention for HIV/AIDS by advancing antiretroviral therapy, gene therapy, immunotherapy, vaccinology, and microbicides.

Keywords: microbubbles, HIV/AIDS, target drug delivery

1. Introduction

The recent advanced methods of noninvasive delivery of therapeutic agents are effective in gene therapy and molecular biology. Besides the well-known application of microbubbles have been demonstrated an effective technique for targeted delivery of drugs and genes and is also used as contrast agents for diagnostic ultrasound [1–6]. A schematic structure of the biomedical microbubble is shown in **Figure 1**. The size of microbubbles is larger than micrometer but smaller than one hundredth of millimeter in diameter which is equal to the size of red blood cell. Because of its smaller size, it can pass in the microvessels and capillaries throughout the body. In aqueous environment, the microbubbles are unstable and show surface tension effect because of this properly it require the shell and filling material. The gas core of microbubbles gets stabilized by lipid, protein, and polymers [7, 8]. In water microbubbles are miniature gas bubbles of less than 50 microns diameter.

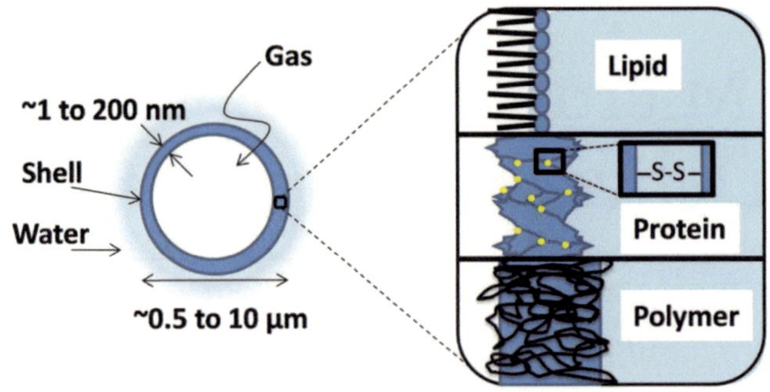

Figure 1.
Illustration describe various shell compositions of microbubbles. The diameter between 0.5 and 10 μm is applied for biomedical use so that it can pass through the capillary of the lung. Microbubbles compose of total particle volume which act as single chamber so that the shell of the microbubble separate encapsulated gas and the surrounding aqueous medium by using various shell materials like lipid with thickness~3 nm thick, protein having 15–20 nm thick and polymer of 100–200 nm thick. Hydrophobic and Vander Waals interactions binds the lipid molecule together and by covalent disulphide bonding the protein molecules get cross-linked so that the formation of bulk like material.

It mostly contains oxygen or air and remains suspended in the water for an extended period. The gas present in the microbubbles dissolves into the water, and the bubble disappears. Incorporation of drug in microbubble includes (1) binding of drug to microbubble shell and (2) attachment of drug at specific site of ligand. In ultrasound-mediated microbubbles, application of high intensity ultra sound can rupture capillary blood vessels resulting in deposit of protein and genetic material into the tissue, ultrasonic rupture of microvessels with diameter 7 μm. Ultrasound forms pores in the membrane of shell. Ultrasound microbubble causes transient hole in the cell surface resulting in rapid translocation of plasmid DNA from the outside to cytoplasm. Low-intensity ultrasound microbubble (0.6 W/cm^2) caused enhanced drug delivery [55]. Microbubbles are usually injected intravenously which is a safe process as compared to the use of conventional method like magnetic resonance imaging and radiography. Microbubble is used in the medical field as diagnostic aids to scan the various organs of the body, and recently they are being proposed to be used as drug or gene carriers and also for treatment in cancer therapy. It is also used to improve the fermentation of soil, to increase the hydroponic plant growth, to increase the aquaculture productivity, and to improve the quality of water, in sewage treatment.

2. Compositions and physicochemical properties of microbubbles

2.1 Protein as stabilizing agent in formation of microbubbles

Albumin-shelled microbubbles were a pioneering formulation used in contrast ultrasound imaging. For perfusion in capillary and microvessels, albumin-shelled microbubbles are very effective. The size of albumin-shelled microbubbles ranges from 1 to 15 μm in diameter in 7×10^8 microbubbles/mL which is stable for 2 years. To formulate albumin-coated microbubbles by sonication method, 5% w/v human serum albumin with air is required and encapsulated within 15 nm thick shell of aggregated albumin. For better encapsulation process, the denaturation of albumin by heating is essential [9, 10]. The albumin shell is held together through disulfide bonds between cysteine residues formed during cavitation [11]. Covalent cross-linking may explain the relative rigidity of albumin shells observed during ultrasonic insonification [12]. Apart from albumin, several proteins are used to coat microbubbles.

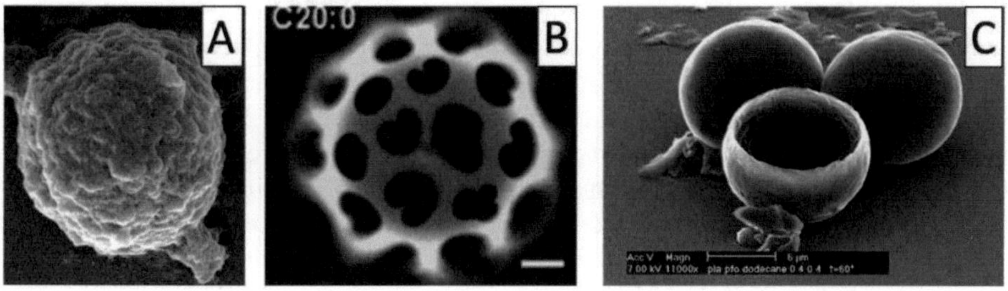

Figure 2.
Microbubble shell morphologies. (A) A lysozyme protein microbubble imaged with SEM (Calaveri et al. (13)). The microbubble diameter is roughly 1 μm. (B) A diC20:0 phospholipid microbubble imaged with fluorescence microscopy taken from Borden et al. Scale bar denotes 20 μm. (C) A PLA-PFO polymer microbubble imaged with SEM.

The proteins which are amphipathic in nature are highly surface-active. In most of the proteins, the disulfide bridge between two thiol groups is present. Cavalieri and co-workers prepared microbubbles by using lysozyme which retain their enzymatic activity for several months and found to be stable [13]. Korpanty et al. [14] developed microbubble by incorporating avidin into albumin shell. **Figure 2A** illustrates targeting vascular endothelium in biotin-mediated coupling of antibodies.

2.2 Surfactant as stabilizing agent in formation of microbubbles

SPAN-40 and TWEEN-40 are used as stabilizing agent in the preparation of microbubbles [15, 16]. For the formation of stable microbubbles, the SPAN/TWEEN solution was sonicated in the presence of air. For maximum film stability, a Langmuir trough was used in the ratio of SPAN to TWEEN (roughly 1:1). By using sonicated microbubbles, modified surfactant was formed which was more stable film due to higher collapse pressure on the Langmuir trough [16]. Dressaire et al. recently reported stable microbubbles formed from a blending process at 70°C in 75 wt% glucose syrup, sucrose stearate (mono- and di-ester) formed [17].

2.3 Lipid as stabilizing agent in the formation of microbubbles

For biomedical imaging and drug delivery, lipid-coated microbubbles are one of the most interesting and useful formulations. The lipid shell is inspired by nature, as stable microbubbles found ubiquitously in the oceans and freshwaters of earth are known to be stabilized by acyl lipids and glycoproteins [18].

During ultrasound and sonication technique, the lipid molecules which are held together by weak physical forces form the microbubble shell having property of expansion and compression without chain entanglement. Lipid-coated microbubbles therefore reduce the damping effect on resonance and reseal around the gas core during fragmentation process [12]. Thus, the lipid-coated microbubble itself is a versatile platform technology. An example of lipid microbubble is shown in **Figure 2B**, which depicts heterogeneity and phase separation of phosphatidylcholine and lipopolymers that are typically used to stabilize lipid microbubble [19].

2.4 Polymer as a stabilizing agent in the formation of microbubbles

The term, "polymer microbubble" typically refers to a special class of microbubbles that are stabilized by a thick shell comprising cross-linked or entangled polymeric species. Polymer shells are more resistant to expansion and compression;

therefore during drug delivery, it reduces echogenicity. During insonification polymer microbubbles release gas core which was unstable and rapidly dissolved [8, 20]. In 1990 a new polymer-shelled microbubble was reported by Wheatley et al. [21] in which the shell was formed by the ionotropic gelation of alginate. By using concentric jells of air and alginate solution, the microbubbles were prepared that was sprayed into a reservoir. On plunging into the calcium solution, the alginate was absorbed by the gas/liquid interface and was hardened. To increase the microbubble yield, sonicate the solution prior to spraying. By using the flow rate of air around the syringe needle, microbubble size was primarily determined. The diameters of microbubbles ranged between 30 and 40 μm and were therefore too large for intravenous administration. In 1997, Bjerknes et al. [22] introduced a method for making microbubbles using an emulsification—solvent evaporation method—encapsulated by a proprietary double-ester polymer with ethylidene units. The polymer microbubbles had a diameter ranging from 1 to 20 μm diameter. Optical microscopy and cryogenic transmission electron microscopy (cryo-TEM) were used for the determination of elongated, crumpled shapes of the microbubbles. The polymer shell was typically 150–200 nm thick. Acoustic tests determine a dose-dependent increase in acoustic attenuation. In 1999, Nayaran and Wheatley describe the preparation of microbubbles by using the biodegradable copolymer poly(D,L-lactide-co-glycolide) (PLGA). By using a volatile solid core, the microspheres were made hollow which could be sublimed. Manipulation of the solution viscosity, polydispersity, and shearing rate microbubble size was controlled. The size distribution ranged from 2 to 20 μm diameter. After incubation in serum the zeta potential of the microbubbles became less negative. In 2005, Cui et al. [23] reported the fabrication of PLGA microbubbles by using a double emulsion, solvent evaporation method. Coulter counter determines the size ranges between 1 and 2 μm diameter. Scanning electron microscopy (SEM) is used to study surface of particles so that the smooth surfaces, visible pores, or cavities can be explained. Confocal scanning microscopy explains internal morphology so that a single hollow core to a more honeycomb structure could be explained depending on the emulsification conditions. In 2005, Cavalieri et al. [24] determined a method of coating microbubbles by using PVA. In this case chemical cross-linking of PVA with microbubbles occurs at the air/water interface with a speed of 8000 rpm, so the mean diameter was approximately 6 ± 1 μm. By decreasing the operating temperature from room conditions to 4°C, the shell thickness could be decreased from 0.9 to 0.7 μm. PVA microbubbles enhance the shelf life of microbubbles by several months. This also increases the incorporation capability of hydrophobic drug and targeting ligand in microbubbles. Bohmer et al. [25] in 2006 used inkjet printing and developed a new technique for the preparation of polymer microbubbles. In this method they injected copolymer polyperfluorooctyl oxycaronyl-poly (lactic acid) (PLA-PFO) having a diameter of 4–5 μm as an organic phase into the aqueous solution (**Figure 2C**).

2.5 Microbubbles used as polyelectrolyte multilayer shells

Polyelectrolyte multilayer (PEM) is a modified type of polymer surfactant shell for the formulation of perforated microbubbles. These microbubbles are coated with charged surfactant which acts as a substrate. To absorb oppositely charged polymer, the layer by layer assembly technique is used [26]. Borden et al. [27] used trimethylammonium propane (TAP) which is a phospholipid containing the cationic head group for creating PEM microbubble where TAP serves as shell. Lentacker et al. [28] described multilayer microbubble. The coating material is DNA and PAH which protect the DNA from enzymatic degradation.

3. Types

1. Perfluorocarbon-filled microbubble, which is stable for circulating in the vascular system as blood pool act as carrier.

2. Ultrasound microbubble, when applied over skin surface where it bursts and releases drug. It is use in low concentration. It also increases therapeutic index. It is advantageous for those drugs which have hazardous and toxic effect.

3. Albumin-encapsulated microbubble, which adheres to vessel walls.

4. Phospholipid-coated microbubble, which has a high affinity for chemotherapeutic drugs [55].

4. Applications

1. Microbubbles increase adherence to damaged vascular endothelium. As the viral proteins obtain in immune response within target tissue the use of viral vector is limited in gene therapy. It has been seen that viral vector causes an intense inflammatory activation of endothelial cells [55].

2. Ultrasound when applied over the skin surface bursts the microbubbles which causes localized release of drug [29–32]. This technique require lower concentration of drug systemically and the concentration of drug only where it is needed therefore the therapeutic index may be increased which is advantageous in case of drug with hazardous systemic side such as cytotoxic agents [33].

3. In diagnostic ultrasound, microbubbles create an acoustic impedance mismatch between fluids and tissues to increase reflection of sound which is used in radiology and cardiology for the detection of perfusion and characterization of tissues. Microbubbles not only increase reflection of sound, they also increase the absorption of sonic energy [34].

4. Ultrasound to contrast agents creates extravasation points in skeletal muscle capillaries. High-intensity ultrasound can rupture capillary vessel resulting in the deposition of protein and genetic material into the tissues. Only a small capillary rupture was required to deliver large quantities of colloidal particles to the muscles [35].

5. Ultrasound increases the transmembrane current as a direct result of membrane resistance due to pore formation [36].

6. Ultrasound-induced cavitation may then be used to destabilize the carriers and affect local drug release. Applications of sonodynamic therapy may include tumor ablation and treating vascular disease such as atherosclerotic plaques. To make targeted microbubbles, targeting ligands were developed and were called bioconjugates suitable for incorporation into membranes stabilizing microbubbles.

7. The anchor locks the bioconjugate into the membrane surrounding the microbubble, and the linker gives the peptide-based targeting ligand enough motional freedom to bind to its target (see **Figure 3**). Thrombus-specific

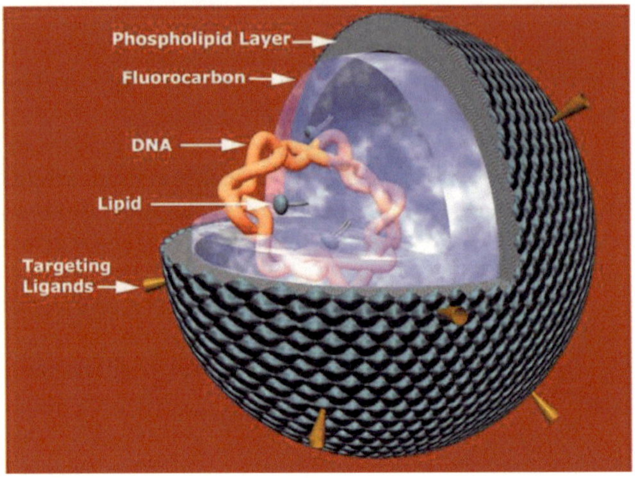

Figure 3.
Liquid perfluorocarbon gene carrier.

peptides, directed to the activated GP2B3A receptor of platelets, were evaluated for affinity to bind to activated platelets by testing for the inhibition of platelet aggregation.

In **Figure 3** the outer surface is stabilized by amphipathic lipid. Targeting ligands have been incorporated onto the head groups of the lipids. The genetic material is stabilized by cationic lipids. Electron microscopy studies have shown that the DNA is condensed as an electron-dense granule within the center of the nanoparticle. The diameter of these particles is about 100–200 nm [37]. There are several advantages to lipid shells. At the air-Space minimized, the phopspholipid's hydrophobic acyl chains face the phopspholipid's gas, and hydrophilic head groups face the water. Thus the monolayer will form around a newly trained gas bubble. Saturated diacyl phospholipids have very low surface tension below phase transition temperature. This is essential as surface tension at the curved interface induces a Laplace overpressure, thus forcing the gas core to dissolve [8]. The microbubble stabilizes at low tension which is achieved by the lipid monolayer [38]. Monolayers of lipids are highly cohesive and form solid-like character because of the attractive hydrophobic interaction between the tightly packed acyl chains and van der Waals [39]. These effect can be effective because the stability of microbubbles during sonication is not dependent on superoxide formation to facilitate disulfide bridging, as is the case with proteins. Therefore, as recently described by Stride and Edirisinghe, lipids are suitable for a variety of manufacturing techniques apart from sonication [40].

In the absence of ultrasound, if the adenovirus was administered with microbubbles using the same model, the author confirmed that plasmid transgene expression can be directed to the heart, with an even higher specificity than viral vectors and that this expression can be regulated by repeated treatments [41]. Lu et al. [42] have also shown that albumin-coated microbubbles significantly improved transgene expression in skeletal muscle of mice, even in the absence of ultrasound.

5. Mechanisms for target drug delivery using microbubbles

Based on the cavitation of microbubbles, two possible strategies for delivering drugs and genes with microbubbles are emerging: the first consists on the ultrasound-mediated microbubble destruction and the second is the direct delivery of substances bound to microbubbles in the absence of ultrasound. Different drugs and genes can be integrated into the ultrasound contrast agent such as perfluorocarbon-filled albumin microbubbles which actively bind proteins and synthetic oligonucleotides [43]. Microbubbles can directly take up genetic material, such as plasmids, adenovirus, and phospholipid-coated microbubbles as these have high affinity for chemotherapeutic drugs.

6. Mechanism by ultrasound-mediated microbubble destruction

Ultrasound facilitates the delivery of drugs and genes. In the insonified field, the presence of microbubbles reduces the peak negative pressure which is necessary to enhance drug delivery. This happened because microbubbles acting as nuclei for cavitations decrease the threshold of ultrasound energy. Microbubble gets destroyed by ultrasound due to the gradual diffusion of gas at low acoustic power, formation of a shell defect with diffusion of gas, immediate expulsion of the microbubble shell at high acoustic power, and dispersion of microbubbles into several smaller bubbles.

7. Mechanism by cavitation of the bubbles

It is characterized by rapid destruction of contrast agents due to a hydrodynamic instability during large amplitude oscillations, and is directly dependent on the transmission pressure [43]. Cavitation of the microbubbles increases capillary permeability and delivery of material to the interstitial tissue. When cavitation occurs, this may impart a ballistic effect to drive the drug from the vasculature into or through the vessel wall. Cavitation events will be intimately associated with the drugs themselves (**Figure 4**) [34]. There are two mechanisms for drug delivery in microbubbles that are incorporation of drug and drug release from these microbubbles.

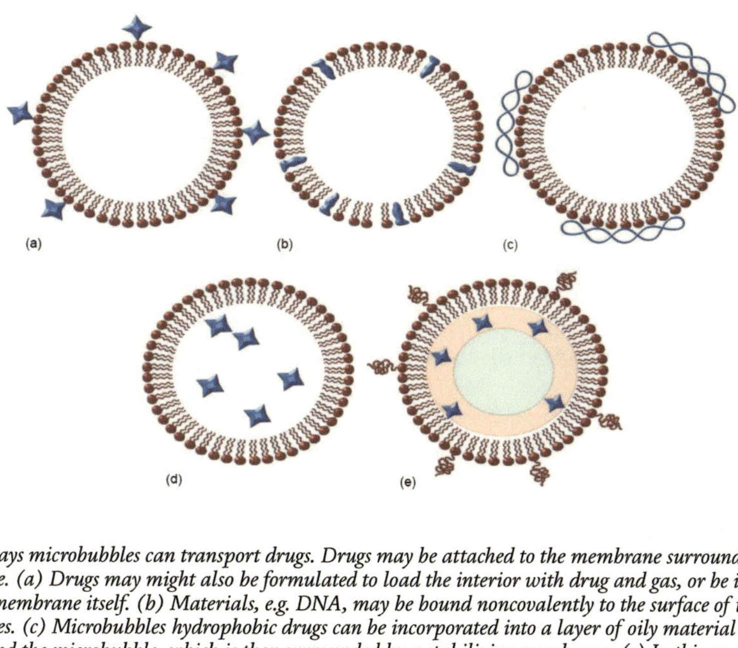

Figure 4.
Different ways microbubbles can transport drugs. Drugs may be attached to the membrane surrounding the microbubble. (a) Drugs may might also be formulated to load the interior with drug and gas, or be imbedded within the membrane itself. (b) Materials, e.g. DNA, may be bound noncovalently to the surface of the microbubbles. (c) Microbubbles hydrophobic drugs can be incorporated into a layer of oily material that forms a film around the microbubble, which is then surrounded by a stabilizing membrane. (e) In this example a targeting ligand is incorporated on the membrane allowing targeted delivery of the drug. Note that although in these examples the stabilizing materials are shown as lipids, but could also be polymeric materials [33].

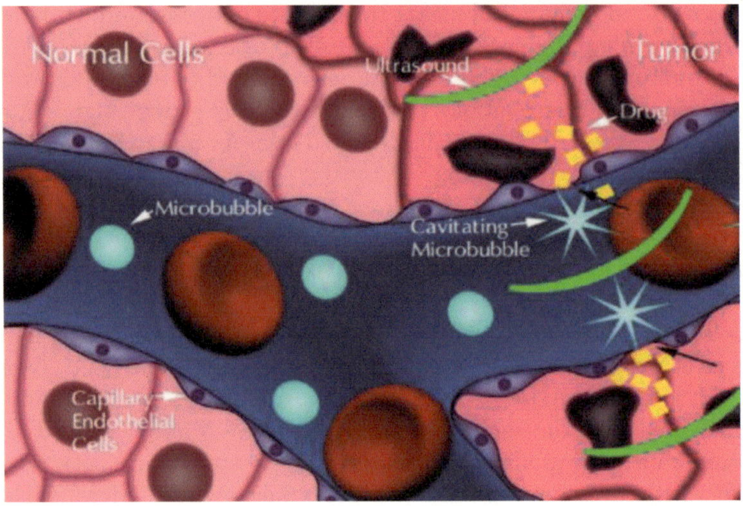

Figure 5.
Drug release from microbubbles by cavitation.

1. **Drug incorporation into microbubbles:** incorporation of drug molecule in the microbubbles in a following way (1) incorporation of drug molecule only within bubble, (2) incorporation of drug molecule within cell membrane, (3) attachment of drug molecule to microbubbles by covalent bonds, (4) attachment of drug molecule to microbubbles by ligand (ex avidin-biotin complex), and (5) incorporation of drug molecule in multiple layer of microbubbles. Microbubbles are able to cross the BBB through above process.

   In **Figure 3** by attaching a targeted ligand such as monoclonal antibody a targeted microbubbles are developed. These are specific for endothelial marker as microbubbles. To assess vascular pathology targeted ultrasound contrast agent are used ex: P-selectin, ICAM-1, GpIIb/IIIa, the αv integrins.

2. **Release of drug from microbubbles:** microbubbles on application of ultrasound undergo a process known as cavitation. Ultrasound causes the microbubble to burst or break. The body fluids begin to insonate on cavitation to create acoustic cavitation. After oscillating microbubbles produces increase small eddy, this increases the permeability of cell membrane and drug passes across the membrane. Microbubbles also release the drug by phagocytosis mechanism. **Figure 5** describe the delivery of drug through fusion mechanism in which the phospholipid microbubble fuse with phospholipid bilayer of cell membrane and releasing of drug or gene into the cytoplasm of cell membrane. By this mechanism the gene get directly transfer to the nucleus of the cell [44–47].

8. Advancements in nano-enabled therapeutics for HIV management

Human immunodeficiency virus (HIV) is a deadly infectious disease worldwide [48–50]. The World Health Organization confirms 0.35 million HIV-infected people. Apart from them, 28 million people are eligible for antiretroviral therapy (ART and only 11.7 million could afford antiretroviral (ARV) drugs. But the ultimate challenge in highly active ART is the elimination of HIV-1 reservoirs from the peripheral nervous system and central nervous system (CNS) [51]. The integration of HIV-1 genome with host genome causes viral latency in the periphery and in brain. However, the inability of ART to penetrate the blood–brain barrier (BBB) after systemic administration makes brain as one of the most dominant HIV infection reservoirs [48]. Recently, dual therapy, i.e., an optimized cocktail of two ARV drugs, has been introduced to manage HIV infection by Kelly et al. [52]. The authors claimed that the dual therapy containing tenofovir (TEF) exerted more therapeutic advantages than triple therapy. Furthermore, the selection of appropriate drug according to the patient condition is very essential because this therapy may reduce virologic efficacy in HIV-infected patient while lowering CD4 counts per high pre-ART HIV-1 RNA level. This report stated that new nanoformulations (NFs) of LA cabotegravir (CTG) and rilpivirine (RPV) may have bright future aspect for HIV therapeutics. This viable dual therapy is useful to manage ART options and performance, which lowers the costs and the globally unmet needs of pill-fatigued and adherence-challenged individuals [52]. The pharmacologic profile of CTG has great potential for the treatment and prevention of HIV-1 infection. This drug has half-life of 40 days and at a low dose showed therapeutic action, so that monthly and bimonthly oral administration in the form of tablet would be enough to control HIV infection [53]. As the significant advancement made in antiretroviral drug for HIV very few efforts have been developed for effective anti HIV vaccine [54]. To cure neuro HIV the inability of effective anti HIV therapeutic agents to cross the complex integrity of the BBB is the major challenge, so neuro HIV is incurable in the brain. Specific receptor binding, focused ultrasound, microbubble assisted focused ultrasound and magnetic field based approaches have been demonstrated to open the BBB for the delivery of therapeutic agents. Due to bigger in size receptor-functionalized therapeutic cargos affect efficacy whereas an externally stimulated approach results in transient BBB opening, which may also allow the delivery of unwanted agents to the brain [55].

Fluoresce activated cell sorting (FACS) is a standard method for diagnosis of AIDS but having high cost and beneficial only in area where large number of HIV patient resides. The second standard technique is Magnetic activated cell sorting (MACS) used for CD4 cell counting. It involves mixing of sample with magnetic beads which get attached to anti bodies. AIDS can be monitored by using the microbubbles which require no expensive equipment and low cost as compare to above methods. In this technique for separation of CD4 T cell lymphocyte from whole blood cell microbubbles are used. By mixing target specific antibody with microbubbles, the microbubbles get float on surface and provide eminent contact between microbubbles and target cell so that target cell attach to microbubbles while non-targeted cell at the bottom side due to gravity [56].

Ultrasound in presence of microbubbles increases plasmid transfusion efficiency *in-vitro*. Microbubbles form pores upto 100 nm by cavitation mechanism which is having short half life. Loading microbubbles with nucleic acid and /or disease targeting ligand may improve efficiency and specificity. Generation of reversible pore in the plasma membrane due to sonoporation increased plasma membrane permeability to marker compounds. Recent studies state that the effect of low frequency 20 Hz by ultrasound on uptake of fluorescent dye calcein having molecular weight 623 Da and radius 0.6 μm into mouse increase cavitation. This data explains that cavitation occur during insonication influence the membrane permeability. Practical and theoretical experiment on microbubble state that the rapid bubble expansion collapse and subsequent shock wave formation can generate shear forces which disturb cell membrane integrity and increased permeability. Further, the geometry of microbubble collapse is itself influenced by adjacent cell membrane like microjet of the surrounding fluid which in transfection medium contains exogenous nucleic acid may get injected in cell [57].

9. Conclusion

Barriers of HIV/AIDS treatment

- HIV is localized in latent cellular and anatomical reservoirs where the majority of therapeutic agents are unable to completely eradicate the virus for the necessary duration.

- The anatomical reservoirs where the HIV get resides are CNS, the cerebrospinal fluid, the lymphatic system, tests, liver, kidney, lungs, the gut and in the macrophage.

- Microphages act as host for viral genetic recombination where it contribute to the generation of elusive mutant viral genotypes

- The other barriers for current therapeutic drug regimens do not fully eradiate the virus from cellular and anatomical reservoirs. In certain cases patient requires to take daily pills which produce patient adherence. These agents have side effect and in some patient resistance develops.

- Current drug therapy can lower the systemic viral load below the detection limit therefore on discontinuation of treatment, there is relapse of the infection occur from the reservoir sites and a potential for resistance develops.

Microbubbles-based drug delivery for HIV/AIDS treatment

- Microbubbles-based drug delivery systems produce complete eradication of viral load from the reservoir sites.

- Micro bubbles containing antiretroviral drugs bind to the CD4+ T cells and macrophages, and reach to latent reservoir of CNS, the cerebrospinal fluid, the lymphatic system, tests, liver, kidney, lungs, the gut and in the macrophage.

- Microbubble-based drug delivery systems deliver antiretroviral drugs in vitro and in vivo.

Microbubble as therapeutic agents

- Microbubbles have average size less than that of red blood cell so it get penetrated into the small blood capillaries and releasing the drug.

- Microbubbles are used as tool for gene delivery.

- Microbubbles can generate strong signal so lower dose of intravenous required and also used in angiogenesis.

Gene therapy for HIV/AIDS treatment

- Gene therapy remove HIV completely from infected cells, as shown by reductions in the cells' overall rate of HIV production. Gene-editing technique.

- Gene therapy based on siRNA has shown promise for HIV/AIDS treatment. Microbubbles platforms for delivery of siRNA for HIV/AIDS treatment are in their early stages but recent work has been met with optimism.

Immunotherapy for HIV/AIDS

- Microbubbles, loaded with both antigen mRNA as well as immunomodulating Trimix mRNA, which can be used for the ultrasound-triggered transfection of dendritic cell (DC).

- DC sonoporation using microbubbles loaded with a combination of antigen and TriMix mRNA can elicit powerful immune responses *in vivo*, and might serve as a potential tool for further *in vivo* DC vaccination applications.

Microbubble used as preventive HIV/AIDS Vaccine

- New approaches are always being explored for development of an effective HIV/AIDS vaccine.

- For delivering DNA various polymer and lipid- based microbubbles have been used.

- Microbubbles encapsulate antigens in their core and cross link to antigen CD4+ and CD8+ T cells. These absorbing antigen allow B cell to generate responses.

- Microbubble vaccines can be given by different route of administration.

Acknowledgements

I would like to express my special thanks of gratitude to my Institute Shri Sachhidanand Shikshan Santh's Taywade College of Pharmacy as well as our principal Dr. C. A. Doifode Sir who gave me the golden opportunity to do this wonderful project on the topic Using Microbubble as Target Drug Delivery to Improve Aids and I came to know about so many new things I am really thankful to them. Secondly I would thankful to Mr. Rafik Shaikh and K.E.M. H.R.C. Pune who helped me a lot in finalizing this project within the limited time frame.

Author details

Harsha Virsingh Sonaye[1*], Rafik Yakub Shaikh[2] and Chandrashekhar A. Doifode[1]

1 Shri Sachhidanand Shikshan Santh's Taywade College of Pharmacy, Nagpur, India

2 K.E.M. Hospital Research Centre, Pune, India

*Address all correspondence to: harsha_20054@rediffmail.com

References

[1] Skyba DM, Price RJ, Linka AZ, Skalak TC, Kaul S. Direct in vivo visualization of intravascular destruction of microbubbles by ultrasound and its local effects on tissue. Circulation. 1998;**98**:290-293

[2] Price RJ, Skyba DM, Kaul S, Skalak TC. Delivery of colloidal particles and red blood cells to tissue through microvessel ruptures created by targeted microbubble destruction with ultrasound. Circulation. 1998;**98**:1264-1267

[3] Porter TR, Iversen PL, Li S, Xie F. Interaction of diagnostic ultrasound with synthetic oligonucleotide labeled perfluorocarbon- exposed sonicated dextrose albumin microbubbles. Journal of Ultrasound in Medicine. 1996;**15**:577-584

[4] Main ML, Grayburn PA. Clinical applications of transpulmonary contrast echocardiography. American Heart Journal. 1999;**137**:144-153

[5] Wei K, Skyba DM, Firschke C, Jayaweera AR, Lindner JR, Kaul S. Interactions between microbubbles and ultrasound: In vitroand in vivo observations. Journal of the American College of Cardiology. 1997;**29**:1081-1088

[6] Unger EC, McCreery TP, Sweitzer RH, Caldwell VE, Wu Y. Acoustically active lipospheres containing paclitaxel: A new therapeutic ultrasound contrast agent. Investigative Radiology. 1998;**33**:886-892

[7] Lindner JR, Song J, Jayaweera AR, Sklenar J, Kaul S. Microvascular rheology of Definity microbubbles after intra-arterial and intravenous administration. Journal of the American Society of Echocardiography. 2002;**15**:396-403 [PubMed: 12019422]

[8] Epstein PS, Plesset MS. On the Stability of Gas Bubbles in Liquid-Gas Solutions. The Journal of Chemical Physics. 1950;**18**:1505-1509

[9] Myrset AH, Nicolaysen H, Toft K, Christiansen C, Skotland T. Structure and organization of albumin molecules forming the shell of air-filled microspheres: evidence for a monolayer of albumin molecules of multiple orientations stabilizing the enclosed air. Biotechnology and Applied Biochemistry. 1996;**24**:145-153 [PubMed: 8865606]

[10] Christiansen C, Kryvi H, Sontum PC, Skotland T. Physical and biochemical characterization of Albunex, a new ultrasound contrast agent consisting of air-filled albumin microspheres suspended in a solution of human albumin. Biotechnology and Applied Biochemistry. 1994;**19**: 307-320 [PubMed: 8031506]

[11] Grinstaff MW, Suslick KS. Air-filled proteinaceous microbubbles: synthesis of an echo-contrast agent. In: Proceedings of the National Academy of Sciences of the United States of America. 1991;**88**:7708-7771 [Pub Med: 1652761]

[12] Dayton PA, Morgan KE, Klibanov AL, Brandenburger GH, Ferrara KW. Optical and acoustical observations of the effects of ultrasound on contrast agents. IEEE Transactions On Ultrasonics, Ferroelectrics and Frequency Control. 1999;**46**(1):220-232. [Pub Med: 18238417]

[13] Cavalieri F, Ashokkumar M, Grieser F, Caruso F. Ultrasonic synthesis of stable, functional lysozyme microbubbles. Langmuir. 2008;**24**:10078-10083 [Pubmed: 18710266]

[14] Korpanty G, Grayburn PA, Shohet RV, Brekken RA. Targeting

vascular endothelium with avidin microbubbles. Ultrasound in Medicine and Biology. 2005;**31**:1279-1283 [PubMed: 16176794]

[15] Singhal S, Moser CC, Wheatley MA. Surfactant-stabilized microbubbles as ultrasound contrast agents: Stability study of Span 60 and Tween 80 mixtures using a Langmuir trough. Langmuir. 1993;**9**(9):2426-2429

[16] Wang WH, Moser CC, Wheatley MA. Synthesis, Characterization And Application of Microbubbles: A Review. Journal of Physical Chemistry. 1996;**100**:13815-13821

[17] Dressaire E, Bee R, Bell DC, Lips A, Stone HA. Interfacial polygonal nanopatterning of stable microbubbles. Science. 2008;**320**:1198-1201 [PubMed: 18511685]

[18] D'Arrigo JS. Stable Gas-in-Liquid Emulsions: Production in Natural Waters and Artificial Media. New York, NY: Elsevier Science Pub. Co; 1986

[19] Borden MA, Martinez GV, Ricker J, Tsvetkova N, Longo M, Gillies RJ, et al. Lateral phase separation in lipid-coated microbubbles. Langmuir. 2006;**22**: 4291-4297 [PubMed: 16618177]

[20] Bloch SH, Wan M, Dayton PA, Ferrara KW. Optical observation of lipid- and polymer-shelled ultrasound microbubble contrast agents. Applied Physics Letters. 2004;**84**:631-633 [Scopus144]

[21] Wheatley MA, Schrope B, Shen P. Contrast agents for diagnostic ultrasound: Development and evaluation of polymer-coated microbubbles. Biomaterials. 1990;**11**:713-717 [PubMed: 2090309]

[22] Bjerknes K, Braenden JU, Braenden JE, Skurtveit R, Smistad G, Agerkvist I. Air-filled polymeric microcapsules from emulsions containing different organic phases. Journal of Microencapsulation. 2001;**18**:159-171 [PubMed: 11253933]

[23] Cui WJ, Bei JZ, Wang SG, Zhi G, Zhao YY, Zhou XS, et al. Preparation and evaluation of poly(L-lactide-co-glycolide) (PLGA) microbubbles as a contrast agent for myocardial contrast echocardiography. Journal of Biomedical Materials Research Part B-Applied Biomaterials. 2005;**73B**:171-178

[24] Cavalieri F, El Hamassi A, Chiessi E, Paradossi G. Stable polymeric microballoons as multifunctional device for biomedical uses: Synthesis and characterization. Langmuir. 2005;**21**:8758-8764 [PubMed: 16142958]

[25] Bohmer MR, Schroeders R, Steenbakkers JAM, de Winter S, Duineveld PA, Lub J, et al. Preparation of monodisperse polymer particles and capsules by ink-jet printing. Colloids and Surfaces A: Physicochemical and Engineering Aspects. 2006;**289**:96-104 [Scopus 87]

[26] Shchukin DG, Kohler K, Mohwald H, Sukhorukov GB. Gas-Filled Polyelectrolyte Capsules. Angewandte Chemie. International Edition. 2005;**44**(21):3310-3314

[27] Borden MA, Caskey CF, Little E, Gillies RJ, Ferrara KW. DNA and polylysine adsorption and multilayer construction onto cationic lipid-coated microbubbles. Langmuir. 2007;**23**:9401-9408 [PubMed: 17665937]

[28] Lentacker I, De Geest BG, Vandenbroucke RE, Peeters L, Demeester J, De Smedt SC, et al. Ultrasound-responsive polymer-coated microbubbles that bind and protect DNA. Langmuir. 2006;**22**:7273-7278 [PubMed: 16893226]

[29] Taniyama Y, Tachibana K, Hiraoka K, Namba T, Yamasaki K, Hashiya N, et al. Local delivery of plasmid DNA

into rat carotid artery using ultrasound. Circulation. 2002;**105**:1233-1239

[30] Chen S, Shohet RV, Bekeredjian R, Frenkel P, Grayburn PA. Optimization of ultrasound parameters for cardiac gene delivery of adenoviral or plasmid deoxyribonucleic acid by ultrasoundtargetedmicrobubble destruction. Journal of the American College of Cardiology. 2003;**42**:301-308

[31] Shohet RV, Chen S, Zhou YT, Wang Z, Meidell RS, Unger RH, et al. Echocardiographic destruction of albumin microbubbles directs gene delivery to the myocardium. Circulation. 2000;**101**:2554-2556

[32] Mukherjee D, Wong J, Griffin B, Ellis SG, Porter T, Sen S, et al. Tenfold augmentation of endothelial uptake of vascular endothelial growth factor with ultrasound after systemic administration. Journal of the American College of Cardiology. 2000;**35**:1678-1686

[33] Villanueva FS, Jankowski RJ, Manaugh C, Wagner WR. Albumin microbubble adherence to human coronary endothelium: Implications for assessment of endothelial function using myocardial contrast echocardiography. Journal of the American College of Cardiology. 1997;**30**:689-693

[34] Unger EC, Matsunaga TO, Thomas M, Patricia S, Robert S, Rachel Q. Therapeutic applications of microbubbles, 160-168 ImaRx Therapeutics, Inc., 1635 East 18th St., Tucson, AZ 85719, USA. European Journal of Radiology. 2002;**42**(2): 160-168 [PubMed: 11976013]

[35] Song J, Chappell JC, Qi M, VanGieson EJ, Kaul S, Price RJ. Influence of injection site, microvascular pressure and ultrasound variables on microbubble-mediated delivery of microspheres to muscle. Journal of the American College of Cardiology. 2002;**39**:726-731

[36] Deng CX, Sieling F, Pan H, Cui J. Ultrasound-induced cell membrane porosity. Ultrasound in Medicine & Biology. 2004;**30**:519-526

[37] Miller MW. Gene transfection and drug delivery. Ultrasound in Medicine & Biology. 2000;**26**(Suppl 1):S59-S62

[38] Duncan PB, Needham D. Test of the Epstein-Plesset model for gas microparticle dissolution in aqueous media: Effect of surface tension and gas undersaturation in solution. Langmuir. 2004;**20**:2567-2578 [PubMed: 15835125]

[39] Kim DH, Costello MJ, Duncan PB, Needham D. Mechanical Properties and Microstructure of Polycrystalline Phospholipid Monolayer Shells: Novel Solid Microparticles. Langmuir. 2003;**19**:8455-8466

[40] Stride E, Edirisinghe M. Novel Microbubble preparation technologies. Soft Matter. 2008;**4**:2350-2359

[41] Bekeredjian R, Chen S, Frenkel PA, Grayburn PA, Shohet RV. Ultrasound-targeted microbubble destruction can repeatedly direct highly specific plasmid expression to the heart. Circulation. 2003;**108**:1022-1026

[42] Lu QL, Liang HD, Partridge T, Blomley MJ. Microbubble ultrasound improves the efficiency of gene transduction in skeletal muscle in vivo with reduced tissue damage LU2003. Gene Therapy. 2003;**10**:396-405

[43] Chomas JE, Dayton P, Allen J, Morgan K, Ferrara KW. Mechanisms of contrast agent destruction. IEEE Transactions on Ultrasonics, Ferroelectrics, and Frequency Control. 2001;**48**:232-248

[44] Klibanov AL. Ultrasound contrast agents for targeted molecular imaging. Bioconjugate Chemistry. 2005;**16**:9-17

[45] Lindner JR. Microbubbles in medical imaging: Current applications and future directions. Nature Reviews Drug Discovery. 2004;**3**:527-532

[46] McCulloch MC, Gresser S, Moos J. Ultrasound contrast physics: A series on contrast echocardiography, article 3. Journal of the American Society of Echocardiography. 2000;**13**:959-967

[47] Van Wamel A, Kooimam K. Vibrating microbubbles poking individual cells: Drug transfer into cells via sonoporation. Journal of Controlled Release. 2006;**112**(2):149-145. [PubMed: 16556469]

[48] Nair M, Jayant RD, Kaushik A, Sagar V. Getting into the brain: Potential of nanotechnology in the management of neuroAIDS. Advanced Drug Delivery Reviews. 2016;**103**(1):202-217 [PubMed: 26944096]

[49] Ruiz A, Nair M, Kaushik A. Recent update in NanoCure of neuroAIDS. Science Letters Journal. 2015;**4**:172

[50] Zhang Y, Yin C, Zhang T, et al. CRISPR/gRNA-directed synergistic activation mediator (SAM) induces specific, persistent and robust reactivation of the HIV-1 latent reservoirs. Scientific Reports. 2015;**5**:16277

[51] Jayant RD, Atluri VS, Agudelo M, Sagar V, Kaushik A, Nair M. Sustained-release nanoART formulation for the treatment of neuro AIDS. International Journal of Nanomedicine. 2015;**10**:1077-1093

[52] Kelly SG, Nyaku AN, Taiwo BO. Two-drug treatment approaches in HIV: Finally getting somewhere? Drugs. 2016;**76**(5):523-531. [PubMed: 26886135]

[53] Trezza C, Ford SL, Spreen W, Pan R, Piscitelli S. Formulation and pharmacology of long-acting cabotegravir. Current Opinion in HIV and AIDS. 2015;**10**(4):239-245

[54] Gautam R, Nishimura Y, Pegu A, et al. A single injection of anti-HIV-1 antibodies protects against repeated SHIV challenges. Nature. 2016;**533**(7601):105-109

[55] Chomas JE, Dayton P, May D, Ferrara K. Threshold of fragmentation for ultrasonic contrast agents. Journal of Biomedical Optics. 2001;**6**:141-150 [PubMed: 11375723]

[56] Chen C, CH-Hsh, et al. Fast sorting of CD4+ T cells from whole blood using glass microbubbles. HHS Public Access. 2015;**3**(1):28-44 [PubMed: 26161433]

[57] CMH Newman1 and T Bettinger. Gene therapy progress and prospects: Ultrasound for gene transfer. Gene Therapy. 2007;**14**(6)465-475 [PubMed: 17339881]

Chapter 7

Nanopharmaceuticals: A Boon to the Brain-Targeted Drug Delivery

Mahira Zeeshan, Mahwash Mukhtar, Qurat Ul Ain, Salman Khan and Hussain Ali

Abstract

Brain is well known for its multifarious nature and complicated diseases. Brain consists of natural barriers that pose difficulty for the therapeutic agents to reach the brain tissues. Blood-brain barrier is the major barrier while blood-brain tumor barrier, blood-cerebrospinal (CSF) barrier and efflux pump impart additional hindrance. Therapeutic goal is to achieve a considerable drug concentration in the brain tissues in order to obtain desired therapeutic outcomes. To overcome the barriers, nanotechnology was employed in the field of drug delivery and brain targeting. Nanopharmaceuticals are rapidly emerging sub-branch that deals with the drug-loaded nanocarriers or nanomaterials that have unique physicochemical properties and minute size range for penetrating the CNS. Additionally, nanopharmaceuticals can be tailored with functional modalities to achieve active targeting to the brain tissues. The magic behind their therapeutic success is the reduced amount of dose and lesser toxicity, whereby localizing the therapeutic agent to the specific site. Different types of nanopharmaceuticals like polymeric, lipidic and amphiphilic nanocarriers were administered into the living organisms by exploiting different routes for improved targeted therapy. Therefore, it is essential to throw light on the properties, mechanism and delivery route of the major nanopharmaceuticals that are employed for the brain-specific drug delivery.

Keywords: nanocarriers, nanoparticles, nanopharmaceuticals, ligand, brain diseases, targeted drug delivery, nanomedicine, route of administration

1. Introduction

Brain besides being a fascinating organ is also known for its complexity. From outside, this delicate organ is protected by a bony structure called skull while internally it is sheltered from noxious substances via some complex barrier systems. These protective barriers impede the treatment strategies adopted for therapeutic purposes [1]. The management of CNS disorders such as dementia, epilepsy, panic disorders, meningitis, and brain tumors greatly depends on the means of attaining higher drug levels at the targeted sites. Physico-chemical properties of the drug molecule mainly dictate its ability to penetrate these barriers and achieve a therapeutic outcome. Thus the ultimate pharmacological response obtained by the potential drug depends on multiple factors like its effectiveness, its uptake or penetration through protective barriers or its ability to bind with specific carrier proteins for efficient transport across the membrane [2]. Among these barriers, blood-brain barrier (BBB) presents one of the types that hinder the transport of the medicinal compounds for treating brain ailments. BBB serves as both physical and transport barrier and is present at the interface of blood and brain. It is a tight junction made of microvascular endothelial cells, astrocytes, and pericytes [3]. Therefore, the development of newer therapeutic strategies is the need of the hour to overcome these transport hurdles.

1.1 Barriers in delivering drug to brain

1.1.1 The blood-brain barrier (BBB)

It is a tight physical junction present at the interface of CNS and blood circulation. It consists of endothelial cells that do not have fenestrations and thus restrict the influx of ions and other solutes into the brain from surrounding blood capillaries. Astrocytes and pericytes surround endothelial cells and thus make it almost an impermeable barrier. BBB allows paracellular transport of small lipophilic compounds (<400 Da) via passive diffusion. This barrier also offers active transport of some hydrophilic compounds by the means of transport proteins (e.g., P-glycoprotein) present at the junction. The transcellular pathway that is used by some compounds to enter the brain includes different mechanisms such as passive diffusion, specific transporters, and transcytosis [4].

1.1.2 Other barriers

Among the primary brain tumors, gliomas are considered the most common. These tumors make a barrier at their early stage termed as blood-brain tumor barrier (BBTB). Although BBTB is permeable at the core of glioblastomas, however, it closely resembles BBB at the peripheral regions. This combination of BBB and BBTB leads to an additional hindrance for drug delivery to reach the glioblastoma cells and thus requires newer drug development strategies to aid drug delivery to the tumor site [5].

Efflux pumps also serve as additional barriers in drug delivery to the brain that are present in endothelial cells lining. These efflux pumps are made up of protein complexes called adherens junctions primarily regulate the permeability of the endothelial barrier [6].

Blood-cerebrospinal fluid also acts as a barrier that limits the free movement of molecules and drug compounds across the brain by strictly regulating the transfer of solutes between the blood and CSF [7].

2. Drug delivery to brain: potential hurdles to overcome

Mainly lipophilic drugs are used to treat CNS ailments and possess a molecular weight below 400 Da and log P between −0.5 and 6.0 [8, 9]. For drugs that are ionized at physiologic pH, it is their unionized fraction that determines the concentration gradient across the BBB for passive diffusion [2]. By considering these facts, a drug should be designed in such a manner that it has optimal lipid solubility so that it penetrates BBB and maintains a therapeutic concentration in the brain. But this is not that simple because only increasing the lipophilicity of the drug molecule via certain chemical modifications may not attain the desired pharmacokinetic effects as it may lead to decreased systemic solubility and bioavailability. It may also have increased protein binding and higher uptake by liver and reticuloendothelial system which ultimately leads to increased metabolism thus leading to diminished active drug concentration at the target site [2]. There are certain drug molecules that penetrate the BBB besides what their lipid solubility suggest. This penetration is attributed to the carrier-mediated transport of these polar compounds present at the tight junctions [10].

3. Nanopharmaceuticals: an approach to achieve brain targeting

Brain targeting is potentially difficult because of multiple barriers. Recent advances in nanotechnology present opportunities to overcome such limitations and to deliver the drug to the brain targets. Nanopharmaceuticals are the relatively newer field that employed "therapeutic containing nanomaterial" with unique physicochemical properties due to their small size (one to several 100 nm), high

Route	Brand	Nanocarrier	Indication	Manufacturer
SC	Copaxone	Glatiramer acetate	Multiple sclerosis	TEVA
IV	DepoCyt®	Cytarabine encapsulated in multivesicular liposomes (20 μm)	Lymphomatous malignant meningitis	Leadiant Biosciences
Epidural space injection	DepoDur®	Morphine sulfate encapsulated in multivesicular liposomes (17–23 μm)	Chronic pain	Pacira Pharmaceuticals
IV	Opaxio®	Paclitaxel covalently linked to SLN	Glioblastoma	Cell Therapeutics
Intratumoral Injection	NanoTherm®	Aminosilane-coated superparamagnetic iron oxide (15 nm) nanoparticles	Local ablation in glioblastoma, prostate, and pancreatic cancer	Magforce
Oral	Avinza®	Morphine sulfate nanocrystals	Psychostimulant	Pfizer/King Pharma
Oral	Focalin XR®	Dexmethylphenidate HCl nanocrystals	ADHD	Novartis
Oral	Ritalin LA®	Methylphenidate HCl nanocrystals	ADHD	Novartis
SC injection	Plegridy®	Polymer-protein conjugate (PEGylated IFN Beta-1a)	Multiple sclerosis	Biogen
IM injection	Invega Sustenna®	Paliperidone	Schizophrenia	Janssen Pharms
IV	AmBisome®	Amphotericin B liposome	Cryptococcal meningitis	Gilead Sciences, Inc.
IV	Abelcet®	Amphotericin B liposome	Cryptococcal meningitis	Enzon Pharma
IV	DaunoXome®	Daunorubicin liposome	Pediatric brain tumors	Under Phase I trial
IV	Doxil®/Caelyx®	Doxorubicin HSPC, cholesterol, and DSPE-PEG2,000	Glioblastoma and Pediatric brain tumors	Phase II Phase II
IV	Myocet®	Doxorubicin EPC and cholesterol	Glioblastoma	Phase II
IV	SGT-53 (SynerGene Therapeutics)	Cationic liposome with anti-transferrin antibody	Glioblastoma	Phase II
—	Cornell Dots	Silica nanoparticles with a fluorophore, PEG-coated	Malignant brain tumors imaging	Phase I

SC, subcutaneous; IM, intramuscular; IV, intravenous; AHDH, attention deficit hyperactivity disorder; IFN, interferon; DSPE, distearoylphosphatidylethanolamine; EPC, egg phosphatidylcholine; PEG, polyethylene glycol.

Table 1.
Marketed nanopharmaceuticals for brain disorders.

surface to volume ratio and flexibility to alter their properties [11]. An alternate definition can be pharmaceuticals engineered on the nanoscale for the therapeutic purpose [12]. Nanopharmaceuticals comprised of different nanomaterial like polymers, lipids, amphiphilic material, metals, inorganic elements, carbon nanotubes, dendrimers, etc., to constitute nanocarriers which can be fabricated in different sizes, shapes, morphology, surface charges and surface groups for the brain-specific targeted delivery of the drug across barriers. Nanopharmaceuticals mediated drug delivery system has the power to penetrate drug moieties across CNS, either passively or actively, and improve bioavailability and therapeutic efficacy of the drug even at a lower concentration. Currently, available marketed nanopharmaceuticals for the brain are mentioned in **Table 1**.

4. Nanopharmaceuticals: brain targeting mechanisms

Nanopharmaceuticals could able to breach blood-brain barriers through various mechanisms. On the simple edge, their smaller size leads to passive delivery of the drugs through transcellular route across brain's epithelial cells or choroid plexus. Criteria for the simple passive diffusion across the barriers are molecular size less than 400 Da, low hydrogen bonding capacity and lipophilicity [13, 14]. Therefore, lipophilic and tailored nanocarriers could deliver the drug through this mechanism.

While extremely hydrophobic molecules like nutrients (glucose and amino acids) pass through active diffusion mechanism with the aid of special transporter proteins. On the other hand, hydrophilic and larger molecules like transferrin and insulin pass through receptor-mediated transport across the membrane [15]. BBB majorly comprised of the endothelial layer which possessed tight junctions; the presence of proteins, namely occludins, claudins and adhesion molecules in the tight junction, make it a tougher barrier [16].

Nanopharmaceuticals are custom-made to surpass the brain barriers through these mechanisms:

- Lipophilic nanocarriers (liposomes, solid lipid nanoparticles SLN) fuse with the endothelial cells and transport the drug through the transcellular pathway or endocytosis. Moreover, nanoparticles provide a sustained drug release pattern in the bloodstream, enabling higher drug concentration to cross BBB [17].

- Furthermore, nanoparticles are functionalized with ligands or specific surfaces to trigger receptor-mediated transcytosis or carrier-mediated transport across BBB. Attachment of ligands like lactoferrin, transferrin, insulin facilitated receptor-mediated transport. Cationized ligands and peptides like albumin cross through receptor-mediated absorptive transport. Nanoparticles surface can be modified to utilize active transport system comprising P-glycoproteins, L-transporters, nucleoside transporter, ionic transporter, multidrug-resistant proteins that transfer the molecules into the brain by consuming adenosine triphosphate (ATP) [17]

Liposomes have been extensively studied and even FDA approved nanocarrier for brain disorders. Surface modulation of liposomes with functional proteins, peptides and polyethers aided targeted drug delivery for brain diseases [18]. PEGylated liposomes and glutathione-PEGylated liposomes evade body's reticuloendothelial system and facilitate enhanced drug uptake across BBB [19]. Moreover, transferrin-modified liposomes [20], TAT peptide-conjugated liposomes [21], glucose-modified liposomes [22], and transferrin-folate bound liposome effectively deliver the drug

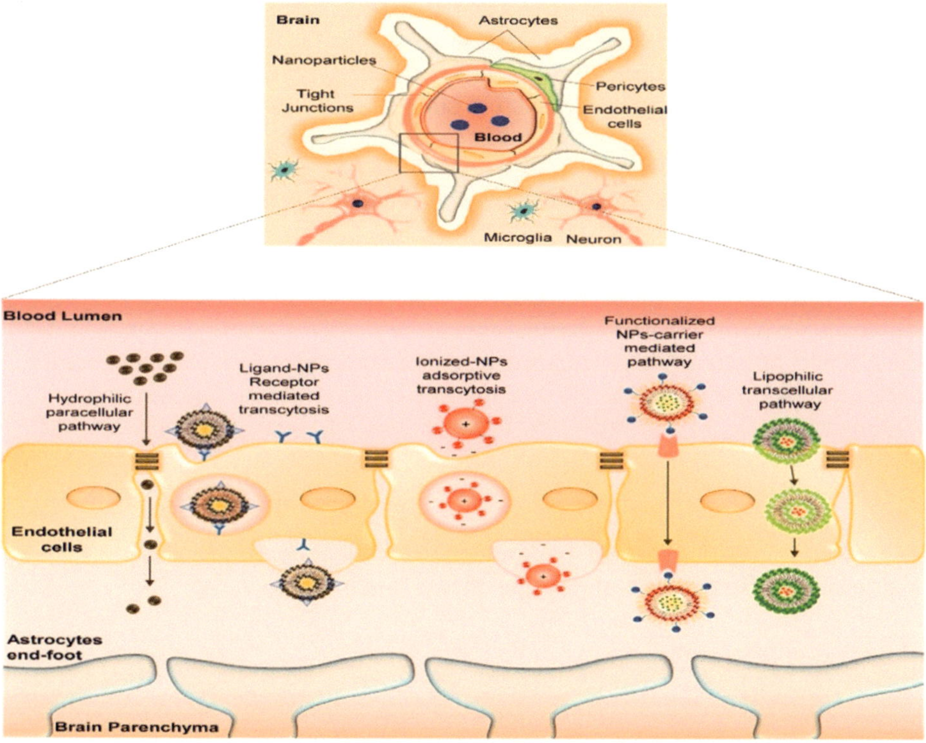

Figure 1.
Different pathways for nanopharmaceuticals mediated transport across the blood-brain barrier (Under Creative Commons Attribution License 4.0, https://creativecommons.org/licenses/by/4.0/) [96].

across the barrier to treat multiple sclerosis [23]. Similarly, transferrin bound SLN and thiamine coated SLN were found to be efficacious in the treatment of cerebral malaria and increased drug uptake in the brain [24]. Mechanisms of transport across BBB are shown in **Figure 1**.

Polymeric nanoparticles accumulate in the brain tissue by both passive and active mechanisms. Chitosan-poly lactic-co-glycolic acid (PLGA) nanoparticles showed enhanced delivery of coenzyme Q to the brain of transgenic mice through absorption mediated endocytosis [25]. In another study, PLGA was coupled with Tet-1 peptide to achieve neuronal targeting of curcumin in the treatment of Alzheimer's disease. Retrograde transportation of curcumin across the barriers destroyed amyloid aggregates and scavenges oxidative radicals in the brain [26]. Similarly, ligand attached polymeric-lipidic nanoparticles like nerve growth factor (NGF) loaded poly butyl cyanoacrylate (PBCA) liposomes considerably deliver the drug across the BBB cholinergic system in the amnesic rodent model [27]. Likewise, inorganic nanocarriers show promising outcomes in terms of brain targeting. Amine functionalized multi-walled carbon nanotubes adopted transcytosis mechanism to pass BBB [28]. A natural substance wheat germ agglutinin-horseradish peroxide (WGA-hrp) was conjugated to gold nanoparticles (AuNPs) and administered in the IM injection into the mice. Results were remarkable in terms of drug penetration across BBB [29].

Dendrimers are the excellent drug carriers; their surface functionalization with folic acid, peptides, aptamers, amino acids, biotin, antibodies facilitated more site-specific targeting. To penetrate CNS barriers, dendrimers were conjugated with transferrin, lactoferrin, D-glucosamine, and leptin for more effective brain drug delivery [30].

Some other nanoparticulate systems like nanoemulsion and nanogel can be functionalized with targeting moieties (transferrin, insulin, peptides) for CNS drug delivery. Nanogels made up of PEG-polyethylenimine (PEI) and N-vinylpyrrolidone/isopropyl acrylamide have been tested to ensure CNS drug delivery potential [30].

5. Nanopharmaceuticals classification on the basis of routes of administration

BBB mediated drug uptake restrictions prompt scientists to investigate drug delivery potential of the nanopharmaceuticals to the brain through various routes. The ultimate objective was to enhance drug penetration across BBB and to reduce disease index. Up till now, the most commonly employed route was systemic administration through Intravenous (IV) injection. Other natural routes like oral, intranasal (IN), intrathecal (IT), intraperitoneal (IP) have been used as well. Some novel strategies like cerebral devices, implants, Ultrasound-guided nanoparticle delivery, osmotic delivery gain much attention in the recent era. Different nanopharmaceuticals are illustrated in **Figure 2**. List of all nanopharmaceuticals delivered through different routes have been mentioned in **Table 2**.

5.1 Oral administration

The oral route is the most convenient, non-invasive and compliant mode of administration. However, brain targeting through the oral route was not investigated largely mainly due to indirect systemic entry through absorption from the gastrointestinal tract (GIT). Harsh GIT environment, slow onset of action, shorter half-life, first pass elimination and reduced systemic absorption hampered drug

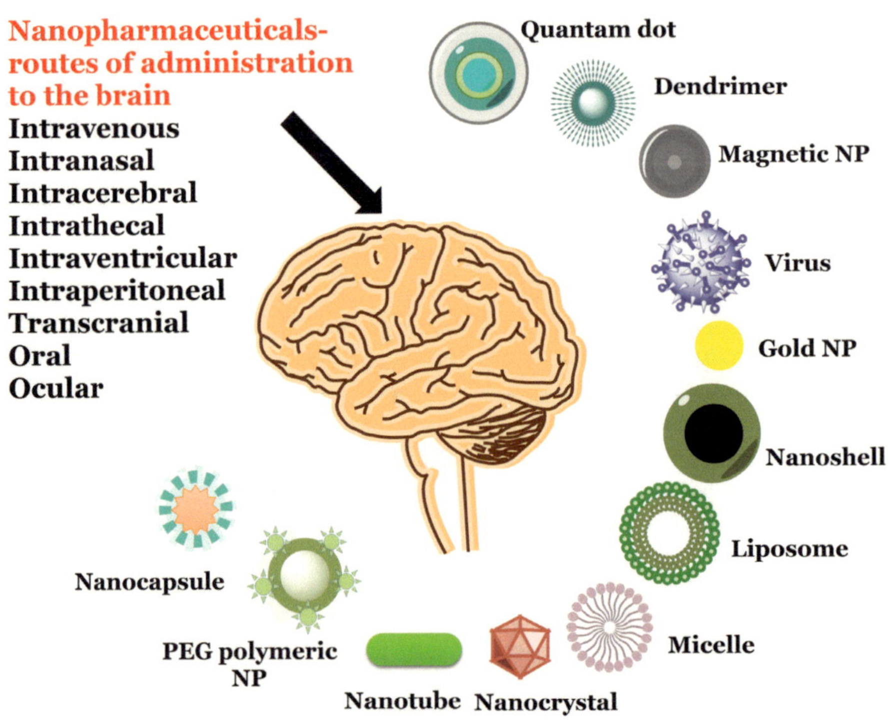

Figure 2.
Nanopharmaceuticals classification on the basis of route and nanocarriers.

DOI: http://dx.doi.org/10.5772/intechopen.83040

Route	Drug	Particle size	Nano component	Active ligand	Indication	References
Oral	Dalargin	~100 nm	poly (butylcyanoacrylate) nanoparticle	Tween 80-PEG 20000	Analgesic effect	[33]
Oral	Indomethacin	~320 nm	Lipidic core	poly (ε-caprolactone) coat	Glioblastoma treatment	[31]
Oral	Saquinavir	100–200 nm	polyunsaturated fatty acids (PUFA), Lipoid-80 and deoxycholic acid		Increase oral bioavailability and brain distribution	[32]
Oral	Estradiol	138.8 ± 4.3 nm	polylactide-co-glycolide (PLGA) nanoparticles	Tween 80 coated	Alzheimer's disease treatment	[34]
Intraperitoneal (IP)	None	220 ± 35 nm	Iron oxide (Fe3O4) nanoparticles	coated with a carbon shell derived from glucose	Brain cells localization	[36]
Intranasal (IN)	Bromocriptine	161.3 ± 4.7 nm	Chitosan nanoparticle	—	Parkinson's disesase	[48]
IN	Clonazepam	15 ± 10 nm	Microemulsion	—	Increase brain/blood uptake ratio	[52]
IN	Nimodipine	30.3 ± 5.3 nm	Microemulsion	—	High brain uptake	[53]
IN	Risperidone	15.5 nm-nanoemulsion; 16.7 nm-mucoadhesive nanoemulsion	Nanoemulsion; mucoadhesive nanoemulsion	—	Schizophrenia treatment	[54]
IN	Diadanosine-dideoxyinosine (dd)	269–382 nm	Chitosan nanoparticles	—	Increase brain/plasm, CSF/plasma ratio	[12]
IN	Rivastigmine	143.1 to 3300 nm	Chitosan nanoparticle	—	Alzheimer's disease	[50]
IN	Venlafaxine	167 ± 6.5 nm	Chitosan nanoparticles	—	Major depressive disorders and anxiety disorder	[51]
IN	Duloxetine	137.2 ± 2.88 nm	Nanostructured lipid carriers	—	Behaviorial improvement in major depressive disorder	[55]

Route	Drug	Particle size	Nano component	Active ligand	Indication	References
IN	Coumarin	100 to 600 nm	methoxy-PEG-polycaprlactone	—	Enhanced brain penetration	[58]
IN	Vasoactive intestinal peptide (VIP)	90–100 nm	PEG-PLA nanoparticles (NP)	—	Protein translocation across BBB	[79]
IN	Sumatriptan	23.1 ± 0.4 nm	Miceller nanocarrier	—	Migraine therapy	[56]
IN	Zolmitriptan	23 nm	Miceller nanocarrier		Migraine therapy	[57]
IN	FITC labeled	5 nm	AuNP	FITC	Brain specific delivery	[80]
Intravenous (IV)	Azidothymidine		Transferrin anchored PEG nanoparticles		Viral infection	[81]
IV	Valproic acid		Nanoparticles		Epilepsy	[82]
IV	Tacrine	35.58 ± 4.64 nm	PBCA NPs		Alzheimer's disease	[83]
IV	Cabazitaxel	24–68 nm	PEG modified Cellulose (Cellax) NPs		Glioblastoma	[84]
IV and intratumoral	Docetaxel/SiRNA	110–150 nm	Peptide modified Cationic liposomes		Glioma	[85]
IV/Intranasal	Catalase	9.5 nm	Exosomes		Parkinsonism	[86]
IV	HCFU	50 nm	Nanogels		Glioma	[87]
IV (MRI)	Curcumin	<100 nm	Magnetic NPs		Detection of amyloid plexus in Alzheimer's	[88]
IV	Sunitinib/ anti-miR-21 oligonucleotide	<190 nm	NPs		Glioblastoma	[89]
IV	Monocolonal antibody (OX26)	300–600 nm	PEG-chitosan NPs		Cerebral ischemia	[90]
Focused ultrasound+IV	FE_3O_4/SPAnH	—	Nanoparticles		Malignant glioma	[91]

DOI: http://dx.doi.org/10.5772/intechopen.83040

Route	Drug	Particle size	Nano component	Active ligand	Indication	References
Convection-enhanced delivery	CPT-11	96–101 nm	Liposomes		Intracranial tumor	[92]
Intrathecal	Fasudil	100 nm	Liposomes		Subarachnoid hemorrhage	[93]
Intracranial	Paclitaxel	3 mm	Nanoscale PLGA implants		Intracranial glioblastoma	[94]
Neural probes	Dexamethasone	400–600 nm	PLGA nanoparticles in alginate hydrogel		Glial inflammation	[95]

PEG, polyethylene glycol; PLA, polylactic acid; FITC, fluorescein isothiocyanate; SPAnH, poly[aniline-c-sodium N-(1-one-butyric acid)] aniline; PBCA, poly(n-butyl cyanoacrylate); HCFU, N-hexylcarbamoyl-5-fluorouracil.

Table 2.
Nanopharmaceuticals administration through various routes.

therapeutic efficacy and bioavailability. Thus, oral drug delivery failed to deliver the therapeutic moiety to the brain efficiently. In this regard, nanopharmaceuticals must possess the properties to bear harsh enzymatic environment, overcome first pass metabolism and efficiently permeate through the intestinal epithelial barrier to reach the systemic circulation.

Scientists developed lipid nanocore surrounded by poly (e-caprolactone) and orally administered to the mice. The concentration of the loaded drug, indomethacin, was successively increased in the brain and efficiently treat glioblastoma in the mice model without causing BBB vessel alteration. This could serve as a basis for safe and effective brain targeting via oral route [31].

Similarly, orally administered saquinavir-loaded nanoemulsion significantly delivers the drug across BBB. Nanoemulsion was stabilized by deoxycholic acid which overpasses first-pass elimination of the drug. The oily phase, polyunsaturated fatty acids (PUFA) facilitates rapid transport to the brain. It laid the foundation for effective brain targeting through oral route [32].

Researchers formulated poly (butyl cyanoacrylate) nanoparticles, double coated with Tween 80 and polyethylene glycol (PEG)-2000 for the oral delivery of the dalargin to the brain. Dalargin is a hexapeptide, anti-nociceptive agent which could not cross BBB. However, its nanoformulation showed promising analgesic effects in the mice model, which demonstrated the potential of the nanoformulation for brain targeting via oral route [33].

Orally administered Tween 80 coated PLGA deliver estradiol successfully to the brain. The therapeutic efficacy in elevating Alzheimer's disease was parallel to the nanoformulation administered intramuscularly [34]. In short, oral delivery of drug-loaded nanopharmaceuticals achieved preliminary success but still need to be further explored in the near future.

5.2 Intraperitoneal administration (IP)

Intraperitoneal administration involved peritoneal cavity of the abdomen. The route is still under investigation. It has an advantage of delivering a larger amount of the drug and it is employed when a vein for the IV injection is not easily located. In addition, it can be employed when animals are not ready for oral administration. However, the route is currently limited to pre-clinical research in small animals and need to be scaled up [35].

Iron oxide nanoparticles were fabricated with the aim to target subcellular compartment of the brain cells. For this purpose, iron oxide nanoparticles with different shapes (round, biconcave, spindle, nanotube) were synthesized and coated with glucose derived fluorescent carbon layer. In-vivo administration through IP route indicated biconcave nanoparticles localized in the nuclei and nanotube-shaped nanoparticles located in the cytoplasm of the brain cells. While the carbon coated surface on iron oxide nanoparticles facilitated attachment of several therapeutic moieties on the nanoparticles for their delivery inside the brain cells [36]. Therefore, the IP route could serve as a major route to deliver the drug across the brain barriers.

5.3 Intravenous administration (IV)

Systemic route including IV drug delivery to the brain involves the receptor-mediated and adsorptive mediated transcytosis. It is the most exploited route of administration for the nanoparticles because of the immediate action systemically and locally by targeted delivery. Polybutyl cyanoacrylate (PBCA) was first used for the synthesis of the NPs intended for the brain. Analgesic dalargin was incorporated in the PBCA NPs with Polysorbate 80 coating and a marked level of analgesia was seen in the animal studies after IV administration of the NPs [37]. PBCA NPs with doxorubicin coated with Polysorbate 80 were studied for their brain delivery in the rats and showed the promising result in 2–4 hours as compared to the uncoated NPs after IV drug delivery [38]. In a similar study, Polysorbate 80 coated PBCA NPs with a size of 280 nm were evaluated for the delivery of Loperamide across BBB following IV injection. Results were quite promising in the *in-vivo* nociceptive studies on mice [39]. Musumeci et al. prepared the docetaxel loaded nanospheres using PLGA and observed the biphasic release of drug following IV administration. An *in vitro* study using a biomembrane model made of dipalmitoylphosphatidylcholine (DPPC) was conducted and confirmed the significant release of the drug across the membrane, making it a potent drug delivery approach for crossing BBB [40]. An *in vitro* study was conducted on brain endothelial cell lines and glioma cells using nanocarrier system made with PLGA/PLA and a detailed sketch of cellular uptake, cytotoxicity and therapeutic efficiency were obtained. Furthermore, the animal studies confirmed the uptake of NPs in the brain following IV administration [41]. In one study, male Sprague Dawley rats were used for establishing the efficacy of curcumin as an anticancer drug with neuroprotective properties. The study group demonstrated that how the nanoparticles can increase the circulation time of curcumin in the body and penetration across the BBB, especially the distribution of NPs in the hippocampus. Half-life and mean residence time of curcumin increased after IV administration of NPs across the BBB [42]. Liu et al. demonstrated the effect of breviscapine loaded PLA NPs in rats after IV administration. NPs with an average particle size of 319 nm were distributed in the liver, spleen and brain. The prepared NPs had longer circulation life because they evaded the RES and crossed BBB [43]. Poly (alkyl cyanoacrylate) NPs can deliver several drugs like loperamide, doxorubicin, tubocurarine, etc., across the brain based on the principle of LDL receptor mediate endocytosis after injection of these NPs into the blood by IV administration. Prior to *in vivo* studies, these NPs were coated with surfactants like Poloxamers and Tween for the enhanced drug uptake by brain blood capillaries [44]. Some of the latest techniques of treating brain disorders include delivery of neurogenic genes, mRNA and siRNA. One such study was reported by Son et al. for the delivery of rabies virus glycoprotein (RVG) labeled disulfide containing polyethyleneimine (PEI) nanomaterial to the brain. *In vivo* studies revealed promising data after the infusion of RVG peptide linked nanomaterial in 6 weeks old male BALB/c mice. [45] MRI-driven targeting of the brain using iron oxide NPs of around 100 nm was reported by the group of researchers. Mice were injected with the NPs suspension and were kept in the magnetic field for 30 minutes. There was 5-folds increase in the accumulation of NPs in the glioma cells in the presence of a magnetic field as compared to undirected NPs following IV administration. This approach can be used as a non-invasive therapeutic and diagnostic tool in the various dimensions of health [46]. However, the associated issues like rapid body clearance through the reticuloendothelial system and unintended organ distribution must be overcome for appropriate brain-specific drug delivery.

5.4 Intranasal administration (IN)

Recently, intranasal (IN) route for the drug delivery to the brain proved to be a reliable and non-invasive mode to cross BBB while possessing the ability to deliver a wide range of drug moieties like smaller molecules, larger macromolecules, growth factors, viral vectors and even stem cells to the brain. The transport involves either olfactory or trigeminal nerve which has a direct link from the brain and terminated in the nasal cavity at respiratory epithelium or olfactory neuroepithelium [47]. The nasal mucosa is the target tissue for the drug administration and possessed features like a larger surface area, porous endothelial membrane, huge blood flow, the absence of first-pass elimination and readily accessible. Olfactory region of nasal mucosa provide nose to brain targeting feature and could able to treat various CNS disorders like depression, pain, Alzheimer's disease, glioblastoma, multiple sclerosis etc. Several dosage forms, sprays, suspensions, nebulizers, aerosols, gel, solutions can be utilized for IN drug delivery [47]. On the other hand, barriers like mucociliary clearance from nasal mucosa, enzymatic degradation and low degree of permeability across nasal epithelium hinder the drug targeting efficiency to the brain. As a solution, nanopharmaceuticals were used which overcome the clearance and other nasal problems due to their unique nature.

One of the studies demonstrated IN administration of chitosan nanoparticle to deliver bromocriptine, a dopaminergic agonist, to minimize motor function disorder associated with prolonged levodopa usage in the Parkinson's disease. Results were promising in terms of motor function [48]. Didanosine-dideoxyinosine (ddI) is an antiretroviral therapy (HAART) and available in oral dosage forms, however, faced extensive degradation and elimination in GIT which decreases its bioavailability. To overcome the issues, dd loaded chitosan nanoparticles were administered through IN route. Results indicated higher brain to plasma, CSF to plasma and olfactory blood to plasma ratios in the case of IN delivered dd nanoparticles. It shows that nanoformulation can be directly delivered to the brain compartment through IN route [49].

Another research group fabricated rivastigmine loaded chitosan nanoparticle for inhibiting acetylcholinesterase in the brain through IN administration. The free drug had severe bioavailability issues and distributed to the non-targeted site with severe side effects when administered through oral or IV route. Here, chitosan nanocarrier and administration through nasal route enhanced brain uptake with higher brain/blood ratio. It further highlighted the role of nanocarrier and route in brain targeting [50]. Similarly, Venlafaxine (VLF) chitosan nanoparticles were administered to the brain through the nasal route for the treatment of major depressive disorders and anxiety disorder with improved brain uptake and enhanced bioavailability [51].

Another study showed microemulsion and mucoadhesive delivering clonazepam, an anxiolytic, sedative, hypnotic, anticonvulsant drug to the brain. The brain/blood uptake ratio of the intranasal microemulsion and mucoadhesive microemulsion were significantly higher than the IV administered microemulsion, indicating the effectiveness of IN route for brain-specific drug delivery [52]. Similarly, the microemulsion was used for the IN delivery of nimodipine to the brain cells. The microemulsion leads to 3-fold more drug uptake by the olfactory bulb than the IV route. AUC ratio of brain to plasma and cerebrospinal fluid (CSF) to plasma were higher after IN administration in comparison to IV injection. Thus, it could be a promising approach to treat neurodegenerative disorders [53]. Risperidone nanoemulsion and mucoadhesive nanoemulsion were administered through IN route for the treatment of schizophrenia. The composition of nanoemulsion included glyceryl monocaprylate as an oily phase, tween 80 as a surfactant and mixture of propylene glycol and transcutol as a co-surfactant. While mucoadhesive microemulsion had chitosan polymer which induces mucoadhesive properties. The nanoemulsion and mucoadhesive nanoemulsion improved risperidone bioavailability, prevent first pass metabolism and bypass BBB to achieve desired drug concentration at the targeted site. The brain/blood uptake ratio and drug transport efficiency were found to be significantly higher through nasal administration in comparison to the IV injection [54].

Furthermore, nanostructured lipid carriers comprising duloxetine was prepared and delivered to the brain via IN route for the treatment of the major depressive disorder. The results revealed prolonged drug release and therapeutic effect as demonstrated from improved behavior analysis after 24 hours [55].

Furthermore, micellar nanocarrier (amphiphilic nanocarriers) of sumatriptan was developed to treat an acute migraine to improve cerebral blood flow. Limitations of the drug associated with oral dosage forms and subcutaneous administration like poor bioavailability, shorter plasma half-life, and hepatic elimination have been resolved to much extent through incorporation in micellar nanocarrier. And increased brain concentration of the drug and site-retention can be achieved via nose to brain drug delivery [56]. Similarly, zolmitriptan-loaded micellar nanocarriers were prepared to target brain serotonin receptors and inhibit cranial vessel inflammation. Micellar nanocarriers were administered through nasal route with enhanced characteristics like lower particle size, higher permeation across nasal mucosa, appropriate flow rate, ability to load hydrophilic as well as hydrophobic drugs, enhanced site-retention and ultimately enhanced drug therapeutic activity [57].

Another polymer methoxy-PEG-polycaprolactone was used to encapsulate coumarin with promising brain penetration and myelin binding properties, while administered through nasal route [58]. Bioadhesive nanocarriers reported in the above studies overcome many hurdles associated with a nasal route like protection of drug against enzymatic degradation, enhanced permeability, and avoidance of mucociliary clearance. However, IN delivery of nanopharmaceuticals should be further improved with targeting moieties and incorporation of cost-effective approach.

6. Alternate routes and strategies

6.1 Conventional enhanced delivery (CED)

Potential brain barriers can be by-passed by injecting the drug directly into the tissues using catheter. Such a direct delivery of therapeutic agent to the target site is termed as conventional enhanced delivery (CED). Many pre-clinical studies adapted CED to infuse nano-formulations directly into the brain [59]. C57BL/6 J mice were used to infuse a 10 μL solution of lipid nanocapsules (LNCs) having an average size of 70 nm into their skull at an infusion rate of 0.5 μL/min [60]. An alternate method for direct infusion was also reported in which drug-loaded micelles were injected by making small incisions on the skull. A foremost shortcoming CED technique is its invasiveness which requires high anesthetic doses prior to incisions, which resulted in the death of the experimental rats [61]. This technique also requires the optimization of certain factors like pH and osmolarity to surpass any brain damage [62].

6.2 Intracarotid delivery

Administering the drug into the carotid artery provides an alternative solution to direct delivery. This direct systemic delivery requires a catheter to directly inject drugs into the bloodstream. In a study, the efficacy of direct systemic delivery was reported almost twice to that of CED in terms of brain damage [63]. IV route is also used to deliver the drug directly into systemic circulation. Ferrociphenol-loaded lipid nanoparticles were infused to manage glioma via the IV route. The outcomes showed that mean survival of the rats was 28 days while mean survival rate recorded foe CED was of 24 days [62, 64].

6.3 Intratumor delivery

Polylactic acid (PLA) and poly-dimethylaminoethyl methacrylate (PDMAEMA) were used to synthesize amphiphilic star-branched co-polymeric nanoparticles for intratumor delivery of the drugs for treating brain tumors. In a study, this system was used to deliver combined DOX and miR-21 inhibitor (miR-21i) into LN229 glioma cells directly. These micelles protected miR-21i from lysosome degradation and the release of DOX to the nucleus, which ultimately decreased the miR-21 expression. This combined DOX and miR-21i delivery surprisingly displayed an anti-proliferative efficiency compared with separate treatment of DOX or the miR-21. The outcomes revealed that this co-polymeric system was a better option for delivering genes and hydrophobic therapeutic agents [65].

6.4 Other parenteral routes

Delivering the drug directly into the brain is another way of treating brain disorders. This local drug delivery has been approved by the US FDA [66]. Intrathecal administration of nanopharmaceuticals delivers the nano-drugs in the CSF. However, this route of administration is most commonly used for anesthetics and neurotic pain [67]. This route is under experimental phases in humans. It includes two different ways of delivering the therapeutic moiety, either by infusion in the intralumbar region or intraventricularly using an Ommaya reservoir placed subcutaneously and connected to the brain with a catheter [68]. Thioflavin-T was delivered by intrahippocampal injection for targeting the β amyloid in the brain using the nanoparticles. The data reported localization of thioflavin-T in the intracellular and extracellular spaces of the brain, which prevented the formation of β-amyloid aggregates in the Alzheimer's disease. This same method can be adapted to deliver the anticancerous drugs as well as other analgesic peptides [69]. In an *in situ* perfusion study conducted on mice, Polysorbate 80 coated PBCA NPs loaded with the tubocurarine were able to cross the BBB after intraventricular drug administration. There was a marked effect on the EEG epileptiform spikes [70]. Intraarterial drug delivery has an advantage over the other conventional systems of drug delivery because of the increased dose delivery at the desired site of the brain. This route can also be exploited for the immun0-targeting. However, this route has some limitations like a dilution of the drug because of cerebral blood flow [71].

6.5 Ultrasound guided drug delivery

Ultrasound facilitated drug penetration through brain barriers is yet another option for safe and reversible targeted drug delivery [72]. In this technique, ultrasound radiations are employed to generate shear stress on the vascular endothelium for a transient and reversible perforation in the BBB which facilitates the nanoscaled drug delivery to the targeted site. It appeared in a research outcome that docosahexaenoic acid binding with low-density lipoprotein NPs can penetrate the BBB by the application of ultrasound sonication. A near IR fluorescent dye examination revealed about 60 times greater accumulation of sonication facilitated drug delivery to the targeted site. The main advantage reported was lack of cytotoxicity or neuronal damage due to pointed ultrasound irradiation [73]. PEGylated PLA nanoparticles delivery to the brain was facilitated via ultrasound-induced perforation. β-specific antibody 6E10 was conjugated on PEG-PLA along with the coumarin 6 and DiR as fluorescent probes to assess the target site accumulation. Ultrasonication facilitated NPs penetration was about 2.5-fold more than the complementary non-sonicating therapy [74]. Ultrasound techniques can be used to aid the enhanced delivery of PEG-b-poly(l-Lysine) coupled with siRNA into glioma cells by 10-fold in conjunction with a newer gas-cored nanobubble [75].

7. Future prospects for nanopharmaceuticals delivery

Another targeted approach to the brain for delivering drugs is through the ocular route. The ocular route has so many advantages like reduced peripheral toxicity and direct delivery of therapeutic moiety in the target site [76]. Ocular and intranasal drug delivery for the brain was compared by a group, in which nerve growth factor (NGF) was used for treating Alzheimer's disease. However, it was found out that intranasal drug administration was more effective and potent for brain disorders and ocular route did not perform well. However, many scientists are working for making the ocular route a success because of it being the compliant and non-invasive route [77]. There has been a huge room for the administration of nanocarrier through ocular route to the brain. Nanocarrier can facilitate drug delivery to the brain because of their size, site-retention properties and enhanced adhesion to the lacrimal fluid. The route can be exploited for the delivery of drugs and genes to CNS by avoiding systemic exposure via nanopharmaceuticals [78].

8. Conclusion

Brain-targeted drug delivery is a difficult matter due to anatomic and pathophysiological brain barriers. The current advances in nanotechnology provide a solution in the form of nanopharmaceuticals, drug containing nanocarriers, to cross the CNS barriers and to target the brain tissue in various disorders. Nanopharmaceuticals' mode of administration into the body is an important aspect, which ultimately effects drug concentration in the brain and drug therapeutic effect. Current chapter highlighted the routes of administration through which nanopharmaceuticals can be delivered to reach the brain. Every route has pros and cons, nanopharmaceuticals overcome the route associated limitations in the delivery of drug to the brain due to their peculiar physicochemical properties and surface modulation. Translation this research area into the clinic still require investigations, as safety is the foremost concern and distribution to other body organs must be eradicated. Moreover, there is a need to control the drug delivery rate when nanopharmaceuticals reach the brain for safer action.

Conflict of interest

The authors declared no conflict of interest.

Author details

Mahira Zeeshan, Mahwash Mukhtar, Qurat Ul Ain, Salman Khan and Hussain Ali*
Department of Pharmacy, Quaid-i-Azam University, Islamabad, Pakistan

*Address all correspondence to: h.ali@qau.edu.pk

References

[1] Dong X. Current strategies for brain drug delivery. Theranostics. 2018;**8**:1481

[2] Begley DJ. Delivery of therapeutic agents to the central nervous system: The problems and the possibilities. Pharmacology & Therapeutics. 2004;**104**:29-45

[3] Sharma U, Badyal PN, Gupta S. Polymeric nanoparticles drug delivery to brain: A review. International Journal of Pharmacology. 2015;**2**:60-69

[4] Pehlivan SB. Nanotechnology-based drug delivery systems for targeting, imaging and diagnosis of neurodegenerative diseases. Pharmaceutical Research. 2013;**30**:2499-2511

[5] Van Tellingen O et al. Overcoming the blood–brain tumor barrier for effective glioblastoma treatment. Drug Resistance Updates. 2015;**19**:1-12

[6] Komarova YA et al. Protein interactions at endothelial junctions and signaling mechanisms regulating endothelial permeability. Circulation Research. 2017;**120**:179-206

[7] Bhaskar S et al. Multifunctional nanocarriers for diagnostics, drug delivery and targeted treatment across blood-brain barrier: Perspectives on tracking and neuroimaging. Particle and Fibre Toxicology. 2010;**7**:3

[8] Bodor N, Buchwald P. Brain-targeted drug delivery. American Journal of Drug Delivery. 2003;**1**:13-26

[9] Levin VA. Relationship of octanol/water partition coefficient and molecular weight to rat brain capillary permeability. Journal of Medicinal Chemistry. 1980;**23**:682-684

[10] Begley DJ, Brightman MW. Structural and functional aspects of the blood-brain barrier. In: Prokai L, Prokai-Tatrai K, editors. Peptide Transport and Delivery into the Central Nervous System. Basel: Birkhäuser, Progress in Drug Research. 2003;**61**:39-48

[11] Bawa R. Nanopharmaceuticals: Nanopharmaceuticals. European Journal of Nanomedicine. 2010;**3**:34-40

[12] Weissig V, Pettinger TK, Murdock N. Nanopharmaceuticals (part 1): Products on the market. International Journal of Nanomedicine. 2014;**9**:4357

[13] Lipinski CA et al. Experimental and computational approaches to estimate solubility and permeability in drug discovery and development settings. Advanced Drug Delivery Reviews. 1997;**23**:3-25

[14] Lu C-T et al. Current approaches to enhance CNS delivery of drugs across the brain barriers. International Journal of Nanomedicine. 2014;**9**:2241

[15] Jain KK. Nanobiotechnology-based strategies for crossing the blood-brain barrier. Nanomedicine. 2012;**7**:1225-1233

[16] Wolburg H, Lippoldt A. Tight junctions of the blood-brain barrier: Development, composition and regulation. Vascular Pharmacology. 2002;**38**:323-337

[17] Saraiva C et al. Nanoparticle-mediated brain drug delivery: Overcoming blood–brain barrier to treat neurodegenerative diseases. Journal of Controlled Release. 2016;**235**:34-47

[18] Micheli M-R et al. Lipid-based nanocarriers for CNS-targeted drug delivery. Recent Patents on CNS Drug Discovery. 2012;**7**:71-86

[19] Rip J et al. Glutathione PEGylated liposomes: Pharmacokinetics and

delivery of cargo across the blood–brain barrier in rats. Journal of Drug Targeting. 2014;**22**:460-467

[20] Koshkaryev A, Piroyan A, Torchilin VP. Increased apoptosis in cancer cells in vitro and in vivo by ceramides in transferrin-modified liposomes. Cancer Biology & Therapy. 2012;**13**:50-60

[21] Wang Y et al. Preparation and evaluation of lidocaine hydrochloride-loaded TAT-conjugated polymeric liposomes for transdermal delivery. International Journal of Pharmaceutics. 2013;**441**:748-756

[22] Xie F et al. Investigation of glucose-modified liposomes using polyethylene glycols with different chain lengths as the linkers for brain targeting. International Journal of Nanomedicine. 2012;**7**:163

[23] Niu R et al. Preparation, characterization, and antitumor activity of paclitaxel-loaded folic acid modified and TAT peptide conjugated PEGylated polymeric liposomes. Journal of Drug Targeting. 2011;**19**:373-381

[24] Gupta Y, Jain A, Jain SK. Transferrin-conjugated solid lipid nanoparticles for enhanced delivery of quinine dihydrochloride to the brain. Journal of Pharmacy and Pharmacology. 2007;**59**:935-940

[25] Wang ZH et al. Trimethylated chitosan-conjugated PLGA nanoparticles for the delivery of drugs to the brain. Biomaterials. 2010;**31**:908-915

[26] Mathew A et al. Curcumin loaded-PLGA nanoparticles conjugated with Tet-1 peptide for potential use in Alzheimer's disease. PLoS One. 2012;**7**:e32616

[27] Kurakhmaeva KB et al. Brain targeting of nerve growth factor using poly (butyl cyanoacrylate) nanoparticles. Journal of Drug Targeting. 2009;**17**:564-574

[28] Kafa H et al. The interaction of carbon nanotubes with an in vitro blood-brain barrier model and mouse brain in vivo. Biomaterials. 2015;**53**:437-452

[29] Zhang Y et al. Transporter protein and drug-conjugated gold nanoparticles capable of bypassing the blood-brain barrier. Scientific Reports. 2016;**6**:25794

[30] Ghalamfarsa G et al. Application of nanomedicine for crossing the blood–brain barrier: Theranostic opportunities in multiple sclerosis. Journal of Immunotoxicology. 2016;**13**:603-619

[31] Rodrigues SF et al. Lipid-core nanocapsules act as a drug shuttle through the blood brain barrier and reduce glioblastoma after intravenous or oral administration. Journal of Biomedical Nanotechnology. 2016;**12**:986-1000

[32] Vyas TK, Shahiwala A, Amiji MM. Improved oral bioavailability and brain transport of Saquinavir upon administration in novel nanoemulsion formulations. International Journal of Pharmaceutics. 2008;**347**:93-101

[33] Das D, Lin S. Double-coated poly (butylcynanoacrylate) nanoparticulate delivery systems for brain targeting of dalargin via oral administration. Journal of Pharmaceutical Sciences. 2005;**94**:1343-1353

[34] Mittal G et al. Development and evaluation of polymer nanoparticles for oral delivery of estradiol to rat brain in a model of Alzheimer's pathology. Journal of Controlled Release. 2011;**150**:220-228

[35] Mujokoro B et al. Nano-structures mediated co-delivery of therapeutic agents for glioblastoma treatment: A review. Materials Science and Engineering: C. 2016;**69**:1092-1102

[36] Chaturbedy P et al. Shape-directed compartmentalized delivery of a

nanoparticle-conjugated small-molecule activator of an epigenetic enzyme in the brain. Journal of Controlled Release. 2015;**217**:151-159

[37] Kreuter J et al. Passage of peptides through the blood-brain barrier with colloidal polymer particles (nanoparticles). Brain Research. 1995;**674**:171-174

[38] Gulyaev AE et al. Significant transport of doxorubicin into the brain with polysorbate 80-coated nanoparticles. Pharmaceutical Research. 1999;**16**:1564-1569

[39] Alyautdin RN et al. Delivery of loperamide across the blood-brain barrier with polysorbate 80-coated polybutylcyanoacrylate nanoparticles. Pharmaceutical Research. 1997;**14**:325-328

[40] Musumeci T et al. PLA/PLGA nanoparticles for sustained release of docetaxel. International Journal of Pharmaceutics. 2006;**325**:172-179

[41] Li J, Sabliov C. PLA/PLGA nanoparticles for delivery of drugs across the blood-brain barrier. Nanotechnology Reviews. 2013;**2**:241-257

[42] Tsai Y-M et al. Curcumin and its nano-formulation: The kinetics of tissue distribution and blood-brain barrier penetration. International Journal of Pharmaceutics. 2011;**416**:331-338

[43] Liu M et al. Pharmacokinetics and biodistribution of surface modification polymeric nanoparticles. Archives of Pharmacal Research. 2008;**31**:547-554

[44] Kreuter J. Influence of the surface properties on nanoparticle-mediated transport of drugs to the brain. Journal of Nanoscience and Nanotechnology. 2004;**4**:484-488

[45] Son S et al. A brain-targeted rabies virus glycoprotein-disulfide linked PEI nanocarrier for delivery of neurogenic microRNA. Biomaterials. 2011;**32**:4968-4975

[46] Chertok B et al. Iron oxide nanoparticles as a drug delivery vehicle for MRI monitored magnetic targeting of brain tumors. Biomaterials. 2008;**29**:487-496

[47] Mittal D et al. Insights into direct nose to brain delivery: Current status and future perspective. Drug Delivery. 2014;**21**:75-86

[48] Md S et al. Bromocriptine loaded chitosan nanoparticles intended for direct nose to brain delivery: Pharmacodynamic, pharmacokinetic and scintigraphy study in mice model. European Journal of Pharmaceutical Sciences. 2013;**48**:393-405

[49] Al-Ghananeem AM et al. Intranasal drug delivery of didanosine-loaded chitosan nanoparticles for brain targeting; an attractive route against infections caused by AIDS viruses. Journal of Drug Targeting. 2010;**18**:381-388

[50] Fazil M et al. Development and evaluation of rivastigmine loaded chitosan nanoparticles for brain targeting. European Journal of Pharmaceutical Sciences. 2012;**47**:6-15

[51] Haque S et al. Venlafaxine loaded chitosan NPs for brain targeting: Pharmacokinetic and pharmacodynamic evaluation. Carbohydrate Polymers. 2012;**89**:72-79. DOI: 10.1016/J.CARBPOL.2012.02.051

[52] Vyas TK et al. Preliminary brain-targeting studies on intranasal mucoadhesive microemulsions of sumatriptan. AAPS PharmSci Tech Journal. 2006;**7**:E49-E57. DOI: 10.1208/PT070108

[53] Zhang Q et al. Preparation of nimodipine-loaded microemulsion for

intranasal delivery and evaluation on the targeting efficiency to the brain. International Journal of Pharmaceutics. 2004;**275**:85-96. DOI: 10.1016/J.IJPHARM.2004.01.039

[54] Kumar M et al. Intranasal nanoemulsion based brain targeting drug delivery system of risperidone. International Journal of Pharmaceutics. 2008;**358**:285-291. DOI: 10.1016/J.IJPHARM.2008.03.029

[55] Alam MI et al. Intranasal administration of nanostructured lipid carriers containing CNS acting drug: Pharmacodynamic studies and estimation in blood and brain. Journal of Psychiatric Research. 2012;**46**:1133-1138. DOI: 10.1016/J.JPSYCHIRES.2012.05.014

[56] Jain R et al. Formulation and evaluation of novel micellar nanocarrier for nasal delivery of sumatriptan. Nanomedicine. 2010;**5**:575-587. DOI: 10.2217/NNM.10.28

[57] Jain R et al. Micellar Nanocarriers: Potential nose-to-brain delivery of zolmitriptan as novel migraine therapy. Pharmaceutical Research. 2010;**27**:655-664. DOI: 10.1007/s11095-009-0041-x

[58] Kanazawa T. Brain delivery of small interfering ribonucleic acid and drugs through intranasal administration with nano-sized polymer micelles. Medical Devices (Auckland, NZ). 2015;**8**:57-64. DOI: 10.2147/MDER.S70856

[59] Allard E et al. Local delivery of ferrociphenol lipid nanocapsules followed by external radiotherapy as a synergistic treatment against intracranial 9L glioma xenograft. Pharmaceutical Research. 2010;**27**:56

[60] Lollo G et al. Development of multifunctional lipid nanocapsules for the co-delivery of paclitaxel and CpG-ODN in the treatment of glioblastoma. International Journal of Pharmaceutics. 2015;**495**:972-980

[61] Corem-Salkmon E et al. Convection-enhanced delivery of methotrexate-loaded maghemite nanoparticles. International Journal of Nanomedicine. 2011;**6**:1595

[62] Huynh NT et al. Administration-dependent efficacy of ferrociphenol lipid nanocapsules for the treatment of intracranial 9L rat gliosarcoma. International Journal of Pharmaceutics. 2012;**423**:55-62

[63] Laine A-L et al. Brain tumour targeting strategies via coated ferrociphenol lipid nanocapsules. European Journal of Pharmaceutics and Biopharmaceutics. 2012;**81**:690-693

[64] Huynh NT et al. Treatment of 9L gliosarcoma in rats by ferrociphenol-loaded lipid nanocapsules based on a passive targeting strategy via the EPR effect. Pharmaceutical Research. 2011;**28**:3189-3198

[65] Qian X et al. Star-branched amphiphilic PLA-b-PDMAEMA copolymers for co-delivery of miR-21 inhibitor and doxorubicin to treat glioma. Biomaterials. 2014;**35**:2322-2335

[66] Guerin C et al. Recent advances in brain tumor therapy: Local intracerebral drug delivery by polymers. Investigational New Drugs. 2004;**22**:27-37

[67] Hwang SR, Kim K. Nano-enabled delivery systems across the blood-brain barrier. Archives of Pharmacal Research. 2014;**37**:24-30

[68] Bleyer WA et al. The Ommaya reservoir. Newly recognized complications and recommendations for insertion and use. Cancer. 1978;**41**:2431-2437

[69] Härtig W et al. Electron microscopic analysis of nanoparticles delivering thioflavin-T after intrahippocampal injection in mouse: Implications for

targeting β-amyloid in Alzheimer's disease. Neuroscience Letters. 2003;**338**:174-176

[70] Alyautdin R et al. Significant entry of tubocurarine into the brain of rats by adsorption to polysorbate 80-coated polybutylcyanoacrylate nanoparticles: An in situ brain perfusion study. Journal of Microencapsulation. 1998;**15**:67-74

[71] Joshi S, Emala CW, Pile-Spellman J. Intra-arterial drug delivery: A concise review. Journal of Neurosurgical Anesthesiology. 2007;**19**:111-119

[72] Yang HW et al. Non-invasive synergistic treatment of brain tumors by targeted chemotherapeutic delivery and amplified focused ultrasound-hyperthermia using magnetic nanographene oxide. Advanced Materials. 2013;**25**:3605-3611

[73] Mulik RS et al. Localized delivery of low-density lipoprotein docosahexaenoic acid nanoparticles to the rat brain using focused ultrasound. Biomaterials. 2016;**83**:257-268

[74] Yao L et al. Facilitated brain delivery of poly (ethylene glycol)-poly (lactic acid) nanoparticles by microbubble-enhanced unfocused ultrasound. Biomaterials. 2014;**35**:3384-3395

[75] Yin T et al. Ultrasound-sensitive siRNA-loaded nanobubbles formed by hetero-assembly of polymeric micelles and liposomes and their therapeutic effect in gliomas. Biomaterials. 2013;**34**:4532-4543

[76] Thakur S, Sharma P, Malviya R. Review: Recent strategies involved in brain targeting through ocular route-patents and application. Annals of Pharmacology and Pharmaceutics. 2017;**2**(8):1043

[77] Capsoni S et al. Delivery of NGF to the brain: Intranasal versus ocular administration in anti-NGF transgenic mice. Journal of Alzheimer's Disease. 2009;**16**:371-388

[78] Abdulrazik M. Method for central nervous system targeting through the ocular route of drug delivery. Google Patents. 2003

[79] Gao X et al. Brain delivery of vasoactive intestinal peptide enhanced with the nanoparticles conjugated with wheat germ agglutinin following intranasal administration. Journal of Controlled Release. 2007;**121**:156-167. DOI: 10.1016/J.JCONREL.2007.05.026

[80] Raliya R et al. Non-invasive aerosol delivery and transport of gold nanoparticles to the brain. Scientific Reports. 2017;7:44718. DOI: 10.1038/SREP44718 Available from: HTTPS://WWW.NATURE.COM/ARTICLES/SREP44718#SUPPLEMENTARY-INFORMATION

[81] Mishra V et al. Targeted brain delivery of AZT via transferrin anchored pegylated albumin nanoparticles. Journal of Drug Targeting. 2006;**14**:45-53

[82] Darius J et al. Influence of nanoparticles on the brain-to-serum distribution and the metabolism of valproic acid in mice. Journal of Pharmacy and Pharmacology. 2000;**52**:1043-1047

[83] Wilson B et al. Targeted delivery of tacrine into the brain with polysorbate 80-coated poly (n-butylcyanoacrylate) nanoparticles. European Journal of Pharmaceutics and Biopharmaceutics. 2008;**70**:75-84

[84] Bteich J et al. A novel nanoparticle formulation derived from carboxymethyl-cellulose, polyethylene glycol and cabazitaxel for chemotherapy delivery to the

brain. Bioconjugate Chemistry. 2018;**29**(6):2009-2020

[85] Yang Z-Z et al. Tumor-targeting dual peptides-modified cationic liposomes for delivery of siRNA and docetaxel to gliomas. Biomaterials. 2014;**35**:5226-5239

[86] Haney MJ et al. Exosomes as drug delivery vehicles for Parkinson's disease therapy. Journal of Controlled Release. 2015;**207**:18-30

[87] Soni S et al. Delivery of hydrophobised 5-fluorouracil derivative to brain tissue through intravenous route using surface modified nanogels. Journal of Drug Targeting. 2006;**14**:87-95

[88] Cheng KK et al. Curcumin-conjugated magnetic nanoparticles for detecting amyloid plaques in Alzheimer's disease mice using magnetic resonance imaging (MRI). Biomaterials. 2015;**44**:155-172

[89] Costa PM et al. MiRNA-21 silencing mediated by tumor-targeted nanoparticles combined with sunitinib: A new multimodal gene therapy approach for glioblastoma. Journal of Controlled Release. 2015;**207**:31-39

[90] Aktaş Y et al. Development and brain delivery of chitosan-PEG nanoparticles functionalized with the monoclonal antibody OX26. Bioconjugate Chemistry. 2005;**16**:1503-1511

[91] Chen P-Y et al. Novel magnetic/ultrasound focusing system enhances nanoparticle drug delivery for glioma treatment. Neuro-Oncology. 2010;**12**:1050-1060

[92] Noble CO et al. Novel nanoliposomal CPT-11 infused by convection-enhanced delivery in intracranial tumors: Pharmacology and efficacy. Cancer Research. 2006;**66**:2801-2806

[93] Ishida T, Takanashi Y, Kiwada H. Safe and efficient drug delivery system with liposomes for intrathecal application of an antivasospastic drug, fasudil. Biological and Pharmaceutical Bulletin. 2006;**29**:397-402

[94] Ranganath SH et al. The use of submicron/nanoscale PLGA implants to deliver paclitaxel with enhanced pharmacokinetics and therapeutic efficacy in intracranial glioblastoma in mice. Biomaterials. 2010;**31**:5199-5207

[95] Kim D-H, Martin DC. Sustained release of dexamethasone from hydrophilic matrices using PLGA nanoparticles for neural drug delivery. Biomaterials. 2006;**27**:3031-3037

[96] Karthivashan G et al. Therapeutic strategies and nano-drug delivery applications in management of ageing Alzheimer's disease. Drug Delivery. 2018;**25**:307-320

Chapter 8

3D Printing in Pharmaceutical Sector: An Overview

Asad Ali, Usama Ahmad and Juber Akhtar

Abstract

The pharmaceutical industry is moving ahead at a rapid pace. Modern technology has enabled the development of novel dosage forms for targeted therapy. However, the fabrication of novel dosage forms at industrial scale is limited and the industry still runs on conventional drug delivery systems, especially modified tablets. The introduction of 3D printing technology in the pharmaceutical industry has opened new horizons in the research and development of printed materials and devices. The main benefits of 3D printing technology lie in the production of small batches of medicines, each with tailored dosages, shapes, sizes, and release characteristics. The manufacture of medicines in this way may finally lead to the concept of personalized medicines becoming a reality. This chapter provides an overview of how 3D printed technology has extended from initial unit operations to developed final products.

Keywords: 3D print, personalized medicines, manufacturing, drug delivery

1. Introduction to 3D printing

Gaining immense interest both in academic and industrial sector is the concept of three dimensional (3D) printing (3DP) technologies. Domains like aerospace, engineering, FMCG, architecture, military, fashion industry, chemical industry, and medical field are by no way untouched by this technology [1, 2]. 3DP has a wide range of applications like tissue design, printing of organ, diagnostics, manufacture of biomedical devices, and the design of drug and delivery systems in the medical field [3, 4]. From the data originated by various techniques like computed tomography (CT) scan and magnetic resonance imaging (MRI), complex anatomical and medical structures according to the need of patient can be fabricated [5, 6]. Replacing and repairing the defective organs like kidney, heart etc. or all together creating a new organ that mimics the same functions as that of original are some additional uses of this technology [7]. This technology is so widespread that its applications include things that are an integral part of human life like clothing, eyeglasses, jewelry, parts of cars, and drugs that can be printed in almost any geometry and shape as per the requirement of the user [8].

In this technology a concept is transformed into prototype by taking help from 3D computer-aided design (CAD) files, hence digitally controlled and customized product can be fabricated [9]. This technology utilizes a bottom-up approach in which layers of materials like living cells, wood, alloy, thermoplastic, metals etc. are placed on top of each other in order to make the required 3D object [10]. Therefore, 3D printing is also known by other terminologies such as layered manufacturing, additive manufacturing, computer automated manufacturing, rapid prototyping, or solid freeform technology (SFF) [9].

In subtractive methodology or conventional method, the product is designed from the bulk substance and due to non-advanced tools used non-standard geometries and objects made from many materials cannot be made with high quality [11, 12]. In contrast to the conventional method, 3DP technology is more automated, rapid and easy to use, customized and sophisticated and cost-effective [13–15].

2. 3D printing procedure

First, a virtual 3D design of an object using digital design software like Onshape, Solidworks, Creo parametric, Autocad, Autodesk etc. is created [2, 16, 17].

↓

This digital model is then converted to (.STL) digital file format which stands for standard tessallation language or stereolithography [2].

↓

Triangulated facets give information regarding the surface of the 3D model that is present in the (.STL) file [2].

↓

The (.STL) file is converted into G file by slicing the design into a series of 2D horizontal cross-sections by the help of specialized slicer software, which is installed in the 3D printer (**Tables 1–2**).

↓

Now the print head is moved in the x-y axis to create the base of the 3D object.

↓

The print head is now allowed to move in the z-axis, thereby depositing the layers sequentially of the desired material, hence creating a complete 3D object [2, 9].

Maximum numbers of 3D printing technologies are compatible with (.STL) file format. Some errors might occur during the conversion of the 3D model to .STL digital file; therefore, software like Magics (Materialise) can be employed to correct the errors during conversion. File formats other than .STL like additive manufacturing file format (AMF) and 3D manufacturing format (3MF) are used as .STL does not have information regarding the type of material, its color, texture, properties, and other features [18].

3. Types of 3D printing technology

3.1 Fused deposition modeling (FDM)

The process involves the selection of the desired polymer, which is melted and forced through a movable heated nozzle. Along the entire 3 axis (i.e., x-y-z), the polymer is laid down layer by layer, which on solidification gives the exact shape as was designed by computer aided design models. Multiple dosage forms like implants, zero-order release tablets etc. that include polymer as a part of their formulation can be made by this method [9, 19–21].

Year	Major development
1980	Dr. Hideo Kodama filed first patent for RP technology
1984	Stereo lithography apparatus (SLA) was invented by Charles Hull
1986	Carl Deckard invented apparatus for producing parts by selective sintering
1989	Patent was granted to Carl Deckard for SLA
1990	Fused deposition modeling (FDM)
1992	First SLA machine was produced using 3D system
1993	3D printing patent was granted to E.M Sachs
1996	Clinical application of biomaterials for tissue regeneration
1999	Luke Massella received first 3D printed bladder which was an amalgamation of 3D printed biomaterials and his own cells
2000	MCP technologies introduced the SLM technology
2002	Miniature functional kidney was fabricated
2003	Term organ printing was coined
2004	Dr. Bowyer conceived the RepRap concept of an open-source, self-replicating 3D printer
2005	First color 3D printer was introduced by Z Corp
2007	Selective layer customization and on-demand manufacturing of industrial parts
2009	Organovo, Inc., announced the release of data on the first fully bioprinted blood vessels
2011	3D printing was applied in gold and silver World's first 3D printed car, robotic aircarft was introduced
2012	Extrusion-based bioprinting for an artificial liver 3D printed prosthetic jaw was implanted
2013	SolidConcepts produced a 3D printed metal gun
2014	Implementation of multi-arm bioprinter to integrate tissue fabrication with printed vasculature
2015	First 3D printed pill was approved by US FDA Organovo announced the release of data on the first fully bioprinted kidney

Table 1.
Historical development in the field of 3D printing (table adapted from Ref. [8]).

3D printing technology used	Formulations	API	Ref.
Semi-solid extrusion (SSE)	Bi-layered tablets (polypill)	Guaifenesin	[30]
	Multiactive tablets (polypill)	Nifedipine, Glipizide, and captopril	[31]
Stereolithography (SLA)	Hydrogels	Ibuprofen	[32]
	Facial mask	Salicylic acid	[33]
Selective layer sintering (SLS)	Tablets	Paracetamol	[34]
	Drug delivery device	Progesterone	[35]
Fused deposition modeling (FDM)	Caplets	Caffeine	[36]
	Tablets	Hydrochlorothiazide	[37]
	Oral films	Aripiprazole	[38]

3D printing technology used	Formulations	API	Ref.
Binder jet printing	Tabular devices	Methylene blue and alizarin yellow (dyes)	[39]
	Cubic tabular devices	Pseudoephedrine	[40]
	Tablets	Chlorpheniramine meleate and fluorescein	[41]
	Orodispersible tablets	Levetiracetam	[42]
Inkjet 3D printing	Implant	Levofloxacin	[43]
3D printing machine	Multidrug implant	Rifampicin and isoniazid	[44]
Inkjet 3D printing	Nanosuspension	Folic acid	[45]
Thermal inkjet (TIJ) printing	Solution	Salbutamol sulfate	[22]
Inkjet 3D printing	Nanoparticle	Rifampicin	[27]

Table 2.
Pharmaceutical preparations that were developed by 3DP technology.

3.2 Thermal inkjet (TIJ) printing

It involves the heating of ink fluid by the help of micro-resistor, thereby creating a bubble of vapor that nucleates and upon expansion forces the ink to drop out of the nozzle. Dispensing of extemporaneous preparation/solution of drug onto 3D scaffolds is an area where this technique can be employed [22, 23].

3.3 Inkjet printing

It is a powder-based 3D printing that utilizes powder as a substrate on which layer by layer different combinations of active ingredients and ink is sprayed which is of varying droplet size that eventually solidifies into solid dosage form [9, 19, 24–28].

3.4 Direct-wise

It encompasses a pattern-generating device that moves as per the guidance of computer-controlled translational stage so that layers after layers are put on in order to achieve a 3D microstructure [29].

3.5 Zip dose

This technology provides a personalized dose in additional to the delivery of a high drug-load with high disintegration and dissolution levels by manufacturing highly porous material [25].

3.6 Vat photopolymerization

It is light-induced polymerization where materials like photopolymers, radiation-curable resins, and liquid are collected in vats, which are successively cured into layers, one layer at a time by irradiating with a light source, thereby providing a 2D patterned layer. This involves techniques such as stereolithography (SLA), digital light processing (DLP), and continuous direct light processing (CDLP).

Depending on the orientation of light source and the surface where polymerization of the photoactive resin occurs, SLA can be divided into two different configurations:

1. Bath configuration (free surface approach)

2. Bat configuration (constrained surface approach) [2].

Advantages of 3D printing in the pharmaceutical field:

1. **Enhanced productivity:** 3D printing works more quickly in contrast to traditional methods especially when it comes to fabrication of items like prosthetics and implants with an additional benefit of better resolution, repeatability, more accuracy, and reliability [7].

2. **Customization and personalization:** One of the pioneer benefits of this technology is the liberty of fabrication of customized medical equipment and products. Customized implants, prosthetics, surgical tools, fixtures can be a great boon to patients as well as physicians [7].

3. **Increased cost efficiency:** Objects produced by 3D printing are of low cost. It is an advantage for small-scale production units or for companies that produce highly complex products or parts because almost all ingredients are inexpensive [46, 47].

By eradicating the use of unnecessary resources, manufacturing cost can also be reduced. For instance, 20-mg tablets could be potentially formulated as 1-mg tablets as per need [19].

4. 3DP allows controlled size of droplets, complex drug release profiles, strength of dosage and multi-dosing [44, 48, 49].

Disadvantages of 3D Printing:

1. In inkjet printing, proper flow of ink can only be achieved with ink that has precise viscosity [50].

2. Ink formulation material should have the property of self-binding but should not bind to other printer elements. In some formulation when the ink does not possess adequate self-binding property or it binds with other elements of printer then the resultant formulation does not have required hardness [51].

3. Rate of drug release may get affected due to binding of ink with other printer materials [52].

4. Medical applications of 3D printing

4.1 Bioprinting of tissues and organs

One of the critical medical issues is the failure of organs and tissues as a result of accident, congenital defects, aging etc (**Figure 1**) and the current resolution for this problem is organ transplant from dead or living donors. However, only few

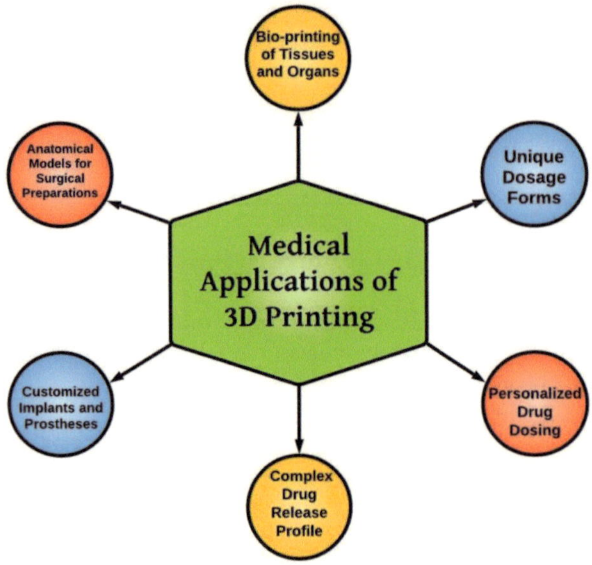
Bio-printing of Tissues and Organs
Unique Dosage Forms
Personalized Drug Dosing
Complex Drug Release Profile
Customized Implants and Prostheses
Anatomical Models for Surgical Preparations
Medical Applications of 3D Printing

Figure 1.
Different medical applications of 3D printing technology.

fortunate people receive organs and the rest die due to donor shortage. Moreover, the procedures for organ transplants are so expensive that it is out of reach of common people. Another problem with transplant surgery is that donors with tissue match are difficult to find [7, 53].

The solution to this problem lies in the fact that the required tissue or organ should be fabricated using the patient's own body cells, which would decrease the risk of tissue or organ rejection; moreover, the requirement for immunosuppressant will also be greatly reduced [7, 54].

In the conventional method of tissue engineering from a small tissue sample, stem cells are isolated, amalgamated with growth factor, and then multiplied in the laboratory. Then the cells are seeded onto scaffolds that direct cell proliferation and differentiation into a functioning tissue.

Placement of cell with accuracy, digitally controlled speed, drop volume, resolution, concentration of cells and diameter of printed cell are some of the additional advantages that 3D bioprinting offers over traditional tissue engineering [2, 54].

Depending upon the porosity, the type of tissue, and required strength, various materials are present to make the scaffolds. Among all materials, hydrogels are said to be the most suitable for building soft tissues [2, 55].

No doubt that organ printing is still in the phase of development but several researches have demonstrated its concept with proof. Scientists have built an artificial ear, cartilage and bone, and heart valve by the help of 3D printers [2, 47, 55]. Wang et al. used 3D bioprinting technology to deposit different cells within various biocompatible hydrogels to produce an artificial liver [54].

As with the increasing interest of researcher and academician and with vast potential of this technology it can possibly unfold new potential therapeutic drugs thereby greatly cutting research cost and time [7].

4.2 Unique dosage forms

Infinite dosage forms can be created using 3D printing. Inkjet-based 3D printing and inkjet powder-based 3D printing are the two main printing technologies employed in the pharmaceutical industry. Microcapusles, antiobiotic printed micropatterns, mesoporous bioactive glass scaffolds, nanosuspensions, and hyaluronan-based synthetic extracellular matrices are some of the novel dosage forms formulated using 3D printing [53] (**Table 3**).

Active pharmaceutical ingredients	Inactive pharmaceutical ingredients
Vancomycin	Glycerin
Ofloxacin	Methanol
Folic acid	Acetone
Dexamethasone	Surfactants (likeTween 20)
Theophylline	Kollidon SR
Acetaminophen	Ethanol-dimethyl sulfoxide
Paclitaxel	Propylene glycol
Tetracycline etc.	Cellulose etc.

Table 3.
List of active and inactive ingredients used in 3D printing.

4.3 Personalized drug dosing

Increasing the efficacy of drugs and at the same time reducing the chances of adverse reaction should be the aim of drug development, which can be achieved by using 3D printing to fabricate personalized medications [7, 26, 53].

Oral tablets are prepared by mixing, milling, and dry and wet granulation of powder ingredients, which are eventually compressed to form tablets; till today, tablets are the most popular dosage form because of the ease of preparation, good patient compliance and accurate dosing and because they are painless. However, no method is available that can prepare personalized solid dosage forms like tablets.

In the traditional way of preparing tablets, drugs can easily undergo degradation if proper guidelines are not followed, leading to altered therapeutic value of the final product. Moreover, these conventional methods cannot be used to prepare customized dosage forms that possess long-lasting stability, novel drug release profile, and detailed geometries [26].

Drugs with narrow therapeutic index can easily be prepared using 3D printing; and, by knowing the patient's pharmacogenetic profile and other characteristics like age, race etc., optimal dosage can be given to the patient [53].

Preparation of entirely new formulation is another vital potential of 3D printing for instance fabrications of pills that have a blend of more than one active pharmaceutical ingredient or dispensed as multi-reservoir printed tablets. Hence patients suffering from more than one disease can get their formulation ready in one multi-dose form at the healthcare point itself, thereby providing personalized and accurate dose to the patient with better or best compliance [26].

4.4 Complex drug release profile

In most conventional compressed dosage forms, a simple drug release profile which is a homogenous mixture of active ingredients is observed. Whereas in 3D printed dosage forms, a complex drug release profile that allows fabrication of complex geometries that are porous and loaded with multiple drugs throughout, surrounded by barrier layers that modulate release, is found [55]. One example is the printing of a multilayered bone implant with a distinct drug release profile alternating between rifampicin and isoniazid in a pulse release mechanism. 3D printing has also been used to print antibiotic micropatterns on paper, which have been used as drug implants to eradicate *Staphylococcus epidermidis* [53].

In a research concerning drug release profiles, chlorpheniramine maleate was 3D printed onto a cellulose powder substrate in amounts as small as 10–12 moles to demonstrate that even a minute quantity of drug could be released at a specified time. This study displayed improved accuracy for the release of very small drug doses compared with conventionally manufactured medications [53].

5. Customized implants and prostheses

By the support of MRI, CT scan, and X-ray and its translation into .stl 3D print files, implants and prostheses of any possible shape can be made [1, 7, 55].

Standard as well as complex surgical implants and prosthetic limbs can be made as per need in time as less as 24 hours. Spinal dental and hip implants have been fabricated so far but their validation is a time-consuming process. Previously, in order to achieve a desired shape and size that fits perfectly, surgeons had to craft metal and plastic pieces and perform bone grafting or use drill machines to modify the implants [2, 7]. This also stands correct in neurosurgery cases due to the irregular shape of the skull whose standardization is a complex procedure.

Some examples of commercially and clinically successful 3D printed implants and prostheses are as follows:

a. First 3D printed titanium mandibular porsthesis was implanted successfully at BIOMED Research Institute in Belgium [1].

b. Dental, orthopedic, maxillofacial, and spinal implants are manufactured by a company named Layer Wise [55].

c. Invisalign braces is another successful commercial use of 3D printing.

By using silver nanoparticles, chondrocytes, and silicon, a prosthetic ear was made out of 3D printing technology that was able to detect electromagnetic frequencies. The impact of this technology is so extensive in the field of hearing aids that today 99% of customized hearing aids are made using 3D printers, because, as everyone's ear canal has a different shape, this technology is able to provide perfect fit for each receiver and, moreover, the devices can be produced efficiently and cost effectively [7].

6. Anatomical models for surgical preparations

In order to have successful medical procedures, knowledge about patients' specific anatomy before medical surgery is essential due to variations in individual and complex human anatomy. 3D printed models have helped extensively in this respect, making them a vital tool for surgical methods [1, 55].

One of the most complicated structures of human body is the head, whose 3D printed neuro-anatomical models are of great help to neurosurgeons. Sometimes, it is very difficult to gain detailed information about the connections between skull architecture, cerebral structure, cranial nerves, and vessels from radiographic 2D images only and even a slight error in the medical procedure can be fatal. Here comes the role of 3D models, which are more realistic and provide in detail comparison and contrast between a normal brain structure and a brain with deformity or lesions, which suggest the surgeons more safe procedures to follow.

- For liver transplant, Japan's Kobe University Hospital had used 3D printed models by using replica of patients' own organ, to find out how to precisely craft a donor liver with least tissue loss [1].
- 3D printed model of calcified aorta for surgical planning of plaque removal was used by surgeons [55].
- To study aerosol drug delivery to lungs, airways of premature infants was reconstructed using 3D printing technology [55].

7. Conclusion

3D printing technology is a valuable and potential tool for the pharmaceutical sector, leading to personalized medicine focused on the patients' needs. It offers numerous advantages, such as increasing the cost efficiency and the manufacturing speed. 3D printing has revolutionized the way in which manufacturing is done. It improves the design manufacturing and reduces lead time and tooling cost for new products. This chapter has summarized different fabrication methods and some notable applications of 3D printing in the healthcare sector, especially in pharmaceutical sciences.

Author details

Asad Ali, Usama Ahmad* and Juber Akhtar
Faculty of Pharmacy, Integral University, Lucknow, India

*Address all correspondence to: usamaahmad.10@outlook.com

References

[1] Klein GT, Lu Y, Wang MY. 3D printing and neurosurgery--ready for prime time? World Neurosurgery. 2013;**80**(3-4):233-235

[2] Gross BC, Erkal JL, Lockwood SY, Chen C, Spence DM. Evaluation of 3D printing and its potential impact on biotechnology and the chemical sciences. Analytical Chemistry. 2014;**86**(7):3240-3253

[3] Chia HN, Wu BM. Recent advances in 3D printing of biomaterials. Journal of Biological Engineering. 2015;**9**(1):4

[4] Liaw CY, Guvendiren M. Current and emerging applications of 3D printing in medicine. Biofabrication. 2017;**9**(2):024102

[5] Rengier F, Mehndiratta A, Von Tengg-Kobligk H, Zechmann CM, Unterhinninghofen R, Kauczor HU, et al. 3D printing based on imaging data: Review of medical applications. International Journal of Computer Assisted Radiology and Surgery. 2010;**5**(4):335-341

[6] Giannopoulos AA, Mitsouras D, Yoo SJ, Liu PP, Chatzizisis YS, Rybicki FJ. Applications of 3D printing in cardiovascular diseases. Nature Reviews Cardiology. 2016;**13**(12):701

[7] Schubert C, Van Langeveld MC, Donoso LA. Innovations in 3D printing: A 3D overview from optics to organs. The British Journal of Ophthalmology. 2014;**98**(2):159-161

[8] Vinogradov P. 3D printing in medicine: Current challenges and potential applications. In: Ahmad NP, Gopinath P, Dutta D, editor. 3D Printing Technology in Nanomedicine. Missouri: Elsevier Inc.; 2019. p. 1

[9] Ventola CL. Medical applications for 3D printing: Current and projected uses. Pharmacy and Therapeutics. 2014;**39**(10):704

[10] Randolph SA. 3D printing: What are the hazards? Workplace Health and Safety. 2018;**66**(3):164

[11] Campbell T, Williams C, Ivanova O, Garrett B. Could 3D printing change the world. In: Technologies, Potential, and Implications of Additive Manufacturing. Washington, DC: Atlantic Council; 2011. p. 3

[12] Hwang HH, Zhu W, Victorine G, Lawrence N, Chen S. 3D-printing of functional biomedical microdevices via light-and extrusion-based approaches. Small Methods. 2018;**2**(2):1700277

[13] Peterson GI, Larsen MB, Ganter MA, Storti DW, Boydston AJ. 3D-printed mechanochromic materials. ACS Applied Materials and Interfaces. 2014;**7**(1):577-583

[14] Anciaux SK, Geiger M, Bowser MT. 3D printed micro free-flow electrophoresis device. Analytical Chemistry. 2016;**88**(15):7675-7682

[15] Wang X, Ao Q, Tian X, et al. 3D bioprinting technologies for hard tissue and organ engineering. Materials. 2016;**9**:802

[16] Roopavath UK, Kalaskar DM. Introduction to 3D printing in medicine. In: Deepak MK, editor. 3D Printing in Medicine. Cambridge, United States: Woodhead Publishing; 2017. pp. 1-20

[17] Patwardhan A. How 3D printing will change the future of borrowing lending and spending? In: David Lee Kuo Chuen Robert Deng, editor. Handbook of Blockchain, Digital Finance, and Inclusion, Volume 2. London, United Kingdom: Academic Press; 2018. pp. 493-520

[18] Gibson I, Rosen D, Stucker B. Additive Manufacturing Technologies, 3D Printing, Rapid Prototyping, and Direct Digital Manufacturing. New York Heidelberg Dordrecht London: Springer; 2010

[19] Katakam P, Dey B, Assaleh FH, Hwisa NT, Adiki SK, Chandu BR, et al. Top-down and bottom-up approaches in 3D printing technologies for drug delivery challenges. Critical Reviews in Therapeutic Drug Carrier Systems. 2015;**32**(1):61-87

[20] Goyanes A, Buanz AB, Hatton GB, Gaisford S, Basit AW. 3D printing of modified-release aminosalicylate (4-ASA and 5-ASA) tablets. European Journal of Pharmaceutics and Biopharmaceutics. 2015;**89**:157-162

[21] Masood SH. Application of fused deposition modelling in controlled drug delivery devices. Assembly Automation. 2007 Aug 7;**27**(3):215-221

[22] Buanz AB, Saunders MH, Basit AW, Gaisford S. Preparation of personalized-dose salbutamol sulphate oral films with thermal ink-jet printing. Pharmaceutical Research. 2011;**28**(10):2386

[23] Meléndez PA, Kane KM, Ashvar CS, Albrecht M, Smith PA. Thermal inkjet application in the preparation of oral dosage forms: Dispensing of prednisolone solutions and polymorphic characterization by solid-state spectroscopic techniques. Journal of Pharmaceutical Sciences. 2008;**97**(7):2619-2636

[24] Sachs E, Cima M, Cornie J. Three dimensional printing: Rapid tooling and prototypes directly from a CAD model. Journal of Manufacturing Science and Engineering. 1992;**114**:481-488

[25] Khaled SA, Burley JC, Alexander MR, Roberts CJ. Desktop 3D printing of controlled release pharmaceutical bilayer tablets. International Journal of Pharmaceutics. 2014;**461**(1-2):105-111

[26] Gu Y, Chen X, Lee JH, Monteiro DA, Wang H, Lee WY. Inkjet printed antibiotic-and calcium-eluting bioresorbable nanocomposite micropatterns for orthopedic implants. Acta Biomaterialia. 2012;**8**(1):424-431

[27] Sandler N, Määttänen A, Ihalainen P, Kronberg L, Meierjohann A, Viitala T, et al. Inkjet printing of drug substances and use of porous substrates-towards individualized dosing. Journal of Pharmaceutical Sciences. 2011;**100**(8):3386-3395

[28] Lewis JA, Gratson GM. Direct writing in three dimensions. Materials Today. 2004;**7**(7-8):32-39

[29] Pharmaceuticals A. FDA approves the first 3D printed drug product. Aprecia Introduces its First Product Using the ZipDose® Formulation Platform for the Treatment of Epilepsy; 2015

[30] Khaled SA, Burley JC, Alexander MR, Yang J, Roberts CJ. 3D printing of tablets containing multiple drugs with defined release profiles. International Journal of Pharmaceutics. 2015;**494**(2):643-650

[31] Martinez PR, Goyanes A, Basit AW, Gaisford S. Fabrication of drug-loaded hydrogels with stereolithographic 3D printing. International Journal of Pharmaceutics. 2017;**532**(1):313-317

[32] Goyanes A, Det-Amornrat U, Wang J, Basit AW, Gaisford S. 3D scanning and 3D printing as innovative technologies for fabricating personalized topical drug delivery systems. Journal of Controlled Release. 2016;**234**:41-48

[33] Fina F, Goyanes A, Gaisford S, Basit AW. Selective laser sintering (SLS) 3D printing of medicines. International

Journal of Pharmaceutics. 2017;**529**(1-2):285-293

[34] Salmoria GV, Klauss P, Zepon KM, Kanis LA. The effects of laser energy density and particle size in the selective laser sintering of polycaprolactone/progesterone specimens: Morphology and drug release. The International Journal of Advanced Manufacturing Technology. 2013;**66**(5-8):1113-1118

[35] Goyanes A, Kobayashi M, Martínez-Pacheco R, Gaisford S, Basit AW. Fused-filament 3D printing of drug products: Microstructure analysis and drug release characteristics of PVA-based caplets. International Journal of Pharmaceutics. 2016;**514**(1):290-295

[36] Gioumouxouzis CI, Katsamenis OL, Bouropoulos N, Fatouros DG. 3D printed oral solid dosage forms containing hydrochlorothiazide for controlled drug delivery. Journal of Drug Delivery Science and Technology. 2017;**40**:164-171

[37] Jamróz W, Kurek M, Łyszczarz E, Szafraniec J, Knapik-Kowalczuk J, Syrek K, et al. 3D printed orodispersible films with Aripiprazole. International Journal of Pharmaceutics. 2017;**533**(2):413-420

[38] Wu BM, Borland SW, Giordano RA, Cima LG, Sachs EM, Cima MJ. Solid free-form fabrication of drug delivery devices. Journal of Controlled Release. 1996;**40**(1-2):77-87

[39] Wang J, Goyanes A, Gaisford S, Basit AW. Stereolithographic (SLA) 3D printing of oral modified-release dosage forms. International Journal of Pharmaceutics. 2016;**503**(1-2):207-212

[40] Katstra WE, Palazzolo RD, Rowe CW, Giritlioglu B, Teung P, Cima MJ. Oral dosage forms fabricated by three dimensional printing™. Journal of Controlled Release. 2000;**66**(1):1-9

[41] Jacob J et al. Aprecia Pharmaceuticals LLC. Rapid disperse dosage form containing levetiracetam. US9339489B2

[42] Huang W, Zheng Q, Sun W, Xu H, Yang X. Levofloxacin implants with predefined microstructure fabricated by three-dimensional printing technique. International Journal of Pharmaceutics. 2007;**339**(1-2):33-38

[43] Wu W, Zheng Q, Guo X, Sun J, Liu Y. A programmed release multi-drug implant fabricated by three-dimensional printing technology for bone tuberculosis therapy. Biomedical Materials. 2009;**4**(6):065005

[44] Pardeike J, Strohmeier DM, Schrödl N, Voura C, Gruber M, Khinast JG, et al. Nanosuspensions as advanced printing ink for accurate dosing of poorly soluble drugs in personalized medicines. International Journal of Pharmaceutics. 2011;**420**(1):93-100

[45] Banks J. Adding value in additive manufacturing: Researchers in the United Kingdom and Europe look to 3D printing for customization. IEEE Pulse. 2013;**4**(6):22-26

[46] Mertz L. Dream it, design it, print it in 3-D: What can 3-D printing do for you? IEEE Pulse. 2013;**4**(6):15-21

[47] Lee BK, Yun YH, Choi JS, Choi YC, Kim JD, Cho YW. Fabrication of drug-loaded polymer microparticles with arbitrary geometries using a piezoelectric inkjet printing system. International Journal of Pharmaceutics. 2012;**427**(2):305-310

[48] Scoutaris N, Alexander MR, Gellert PR, Roberts CJ. Inkjet printing as a novel medicine formulation technique. Journal of Controlled Release. 2011;**156**(2):179-185

[49] Katstra WE. Fabrication of complex oral drug delivery forms by Three Dimensional Printing (tm). Doctoral dissertation. Massachusetts Institute of Technology

[50] Yu DG, Branford-White C, Yang YC, Zhu LM, Welbeck EW, Yang XL. A novel fast disintegrating tablet fabricated by three-dimensional printing. Drug Development and Industrial Pharmacy. 2009;**35**(12):1530-1536

[51] Ursan ID, Chiu L, Pierce A. Three-dimensional drug printing: A structured review. Journal of the American Pharmacists Association. 2013;**53**(2):136-144

[52] Cui X, Boland T, DD'Lima D, Lotz MK. Thermal inkjet printing in tissue engineering and regenerative medicine. Recent Patents on Drug Delivery and Formulation. 2012;**6**(2):149-155

[53] Ozbolat IT, Yu Y. Bioprinting toward organ fabrication: Challenges and future trends. IEEE Transactions on Biomedical Engineering. 2013;**60**(3):691-699

[54] Bartlett S. Printing organs on demand. The Lancet Respiratory Medicine. 2013;**1**(9):684

[55] Lipson H. New world of 3-D printing offers "completely new ways of thinking": Q&A with author, engineer, and 3-D printing expert Hod Lipson. IEEE Pulse. 2013;**4**(6):12-14